YOUR HOMEMADE

HAND

SANITIZER

RECIPES

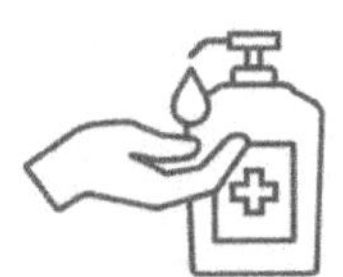

A BEGINNER'S GUIDE WITH EFFECTIVE DIY RECIPES TO MAKE YOUR BEST ATIBACTERIAL GEL, SPRAY DISINFECTANT AND CLEANING WIPES

EMMA KINGS

TABLE OF CONTENTS

16. DIY HAND SANITIZER GEL RECIPES (HOW TO MAKE) 122

17. DIY HAND SANITIZER SPRAY RECIPES 131

18. DIY DISINFECTANT SURFACE WIPES 139

Introduction

Hand sanitizer is a liquid or gel used to reduce infectious agents which are on our hands. This alcohol-based formulation is generally more effective at killing germs and diseases on the hands and is more preferable to hand washing in antiseptic soap and water. They exist in liquid, foam, and gel formulations, something we are going to be looking at as we go further.

Simply put, hand sanitizers are healthy and we are going to be looking at how you can make then for yourself, particularly now that it is needed the most.

When using a hand sanitizer, you have to rub it in your skin till your arms are dried. And, you're to wash your hands first with soap and water if your hands are messy or dirty.

Sprinkle or apply your hand sanitizer on one palm. Rub your hands together thoroughly. Make sure all your hand surfaces and all fingers are covered. Continue to rub for 60 seconds or till your hands are dry. For the hand sanitizer to kill more germs, it can take at least 60 seconds and sometimes even longer.

Making hand sanitizer at home is not difficult or time-consuming. In only a couple of minutes, and using basic ingredients, you can create your own hand sanitizer that will keep you as safe as the products that you typically buy from the store. By learning these recipes, you will see that it is easier than you might think to stay protected. The following recipes will provide you with a variety of ways to make your own hand sanitizer: you can try them all to see which ones you enjoy most. Whether you make a gel or a spray, these recipes are sure to become a staple in your household.

Before you get started, keep in mind that the potency of any hand sanitizer you make is going to matter a great deal. Luckily, this staple item is one that many households already keep in stock at all times. The rubbing alcohol is the main ingredient that is going to protect you, and also come in handy during other emergency medical situations.

If possible, you should aim for an even higher potency when you make your sanitizer. Sticking to a minimum of 75% rubbing alcohol will ensure that you are adequately protected. Using 99% isopropyl rubbing alcohol is what most recipes call for. Individuals who use vodka and whiskey in its place are not likely to end up making a sanitizer that is as effective due to the small percentage of alcohol present in these liquors. Sticking to pure alcohol is always going to benefit you more.

Don't forget to properly sanitize any tools that you are going to use while making your hand sanitizer: it defeats the purpose if you are not hygienic when you make it. Clean your hands thoroughly before you handle any of the ingredients or supplies that you will be using. Having this kind of awareness will get you into better habits while also giving you the peace of mind of knowing that your hand sanitizer is going to be effective. Make sure that you also have proper storage containers or spray bottles, depending on what kind of sanitizer you are making.

Hand sanitizer is a modern purifying drug that takes over soap and water easily. It has good antiseptic properties and incorporates alcohol, which can destroy germs more effectively than the old washing process. Sanitizer comes in foam, liquid, or spray, and several different companies manufacture it in bottles of varying sizes.

It's a fairly new and incredibly handy commodity. Most people bring small bottles or pockets in their luggage to help shield them from germs because they do not have access to sinks. These people are fanatical, putting it on their hands every time they open a door or pass a piece of merchandise.

1. HAND SANITIZER

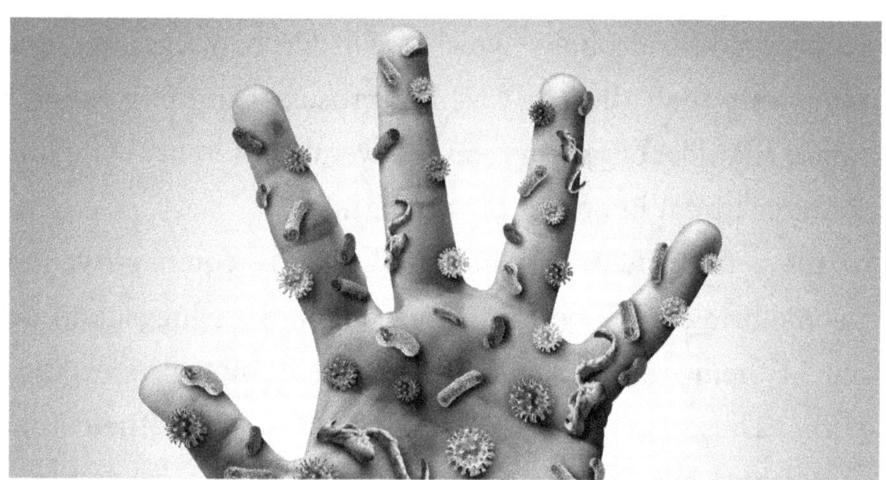

WHAT IS A SANITIZER?

Hand sanitizer is a chemical agent applied to the hands, typically in the form of colorless liquid, foam, or gel to remove bacteria, pathogens, etc. When soap and water are unavailable for hand washing, hand sanitizers are used.

These days, several diseases can be caught by skin contact. So, playing it safe is certainly not an awful thing. Washing your hands with soap and better is the most ideal approach to keep the germs under control. In any case, as we as a whole know, it is not always possible. Wherever we go, especially when we are with the family, it is better to bring hand sanitizer to sanitize our hands whenever we don't have access to soap and water.

There are many kinds of hand sanitizer products you can find in the market. The best are those with 60-80% alcohol concentration as they are very effective in sanitizing purposes and killing germs. Or you can also go for the natural oil base sanitizer with disinfectant properties. Cedar wood, clove, lavender, lemon, pine, tea tree and ylang-ylang essential oils have antiseptic and disinfectant properties. But among these oils, tea tree oil is the most powerful because it also contains antiviral, anti-fungal and antibacterial properties.

Whatever you choose, it is important that the sanitizer has moisturizers to keep your hands and skin from drying. Now, if you want to make sure of the hand sanitizer you and your family will use, you can choose to make your own hand sanitizer. It will save you money plus, you can personally choose the ingredients to use.

BENEFITS OF HOMEMADE HAND SANITIZER

What are the benefits of using a homemade hand sanitizer gel? It protects us from bacteria. These possible microbes live for a short time in our hands, but if we just take them to the mouth, nose, or eyes, we run the risk of catching an infection.

With the homemade sanitizer, the risk is significantly reduced. To this advantage we add these others:

Creating our hand sanitizer saves money and time by not having to go to pharmacies or supermarkets to buy one.

The one prepared at home is free of any preservative because it is made from natural elements.

You can choose the consistency of the gel yourself by putting more or less aloe vera in addition to the aroma when selecting the essential oil.

Remember that once you are going to use the gel, you do not need water. You will only have to apply a small amount and rub both hands well until it has been completely absorbed. You can share your disinfectant gel, but make sure that the nozzle of the dosing container does not touch your hands.

WHY MAKE YOUR OWN SANITIZER?

Some people think that washing their hands is a more effective way to kill bacteria. Hand disinfectant is a complement to hand washing because washing your hands can remove dirt, water droplets, etc. But for bacteria, it is recommended using regular hand sanitizer without soap and water."

It is wise to use a reasonable amount of homemade hand disinfectants when washing your hands. The best antiseptic used in homemade Sanitizers is alcohol, other products such as bleach can irritate the skin.

WHAT ARE THE NEEDED ITEMS?

Creating your personal (or household) hand sanitizer isn't difficult to accomplish and simply involves a few elements:

Rubbing alcohol (or isopropyl alcohol) with a concentration of over 95%, or ethanol

Aloe vera gel (for smoothening out the causticity of the alcohol)

Any good essential oil (this is optional)

The essential factor required to produce a potent, germ-combating hand sanitizer is to abide by a 2:1 ratio of alcohol to aloe vera when adding constituent elements. This is the least possible amount of alcohol required to terminate the majority of germs.

Are Homemade Hand Sanitizers Safe?

The short answer here is, yes - homemade hand sanitizer can be safe and even effective at killing any virus. However, to ensure its antiseptic benefits, sanitizer must be made carefully and properly, and with the correct ingredients. Fortunately, there is a wealth of information about what actually works - and what doesn't. Isopropyl alcohol is the recommended main ingredient, meaning many DIY recipes that are circulating right now may not be as effective as they are touted to be. Others contain dangerous ingredients like bleach, which is not safe to apply to your skin. However, as long as the guidelines are followed, there's no reason you cannot make your own effective hand sanitizer using rubbing alcohol.

It's important to be informed about all the ingredients you use in making sanitizer

OTHER WAYS YOU CAN USE HAND SANITIZER AT HOME

With all the hype about hand sanitizer lately, it's no surprise that some hand sanitizer "hacks" have found their way into pop culture. Here are the top ten most useful ones:

You can use hand sanitizing liquid to clean your makeup brushes and ensure they are properly sanitized. Protecting the skin on your face from germs is just as important as protecting your hands, but other methods of cleaning your brushes might not remove all the bacteria. Simply saturate the bristles of your brushes with sanitizer and rub them gently in straight strokes for at least 20 seconds, then rinse thoroughly with water to remove all the makeup residue. Let your brushes air dry completely on a clean towel before using them again.

Sanitizers will also remove most kinds of makeup stains from your clothes. Rub some sanitizer on the stain and then rinse with cool water. Be sure to do a spot test on delicate fabrics though, to ensure the sanitizer won't damage your clothing.

Thanks to its alcohol content, hand sanitizer is very effective at removing those accidental pen marks from your skin. Next time you smudge ink on your hand, just use sanitizer as you usually would and watch those annoying ink marks disappear!

Some of the ingredients in most sanitizers, aloe vera in particular, are great for soothing irritated skin. If you get an insect bite, swipe on some hand sanitizer to soothe the itch. It will also help reduce inflammation. Just be sure not to put it on skin that's been broken from scratching – that will give you a nasty stinging sensation.

Trying to get rid of that persistently sticky glue after removing a label? Rather than trying to scrape it off with your fingernails, just apply some sanitizer and rub it with a cloth. The sanitizer will loosen the glue and allow the residue to come off quite easily.

One of the most germy, disgusting things we touch (though we don't often think about it) are our mobile phones. Between germs from your hands, face, and all the places you lay it down, your phone quickly becomes a virtual petri dish paradise for germs. Just saturate a paper towel with a pump of hand sanitizer and thoroughly wipe down your phone. Then you can get back to scrolling through social media – more hygienically.

Did you know that smell emanating from your sweaty armpits is actually caused by bacteria on your skin? If you find yourself in a smelly situation with no deodorant in sight, simply wipe down your pits with a bit of hand sanitizer so you can feel refreshed.

More of us endure the annoyance of acne than we would probably like to admit. It always seems to pop up at the least convenient of times – like when you're far from home and out of reach of your arsenal of facial products. If you find yourself in this frustrating situation, try dabbing a small amount of hand sanitizer on the offending blemish. Since acne is caused by bacteria, the antibacterial properties of your sanitizer will help to reduce it more quickly. Don't use this hack too often though, since the alcohol in sanitizer can dry out your skin if you overdo it.

For those of us who are glasses wearers, one of the most annoying things that can happen is getting a smudge on our lenses. Chances are, if you're out and about, you might not have a wet lens wipe or a bottle of lens cleaner with you. But if you have hand sanitizer on hand, it works as a perfect substitute. Just apply a few drops to your glasses lens and wipe it gently with a soft cloth.

Finally, hand sanitizer can also help you keep things clean around your home. From those pesky fingerprints on walls doors and stainless-steel appliances, to scuff marks and marker masterpieces on your walls (for those who have children) applying a bit of hand sanitizer and rubbing gently with a cloth will often do the trick. Just be sure to do a spot test first to avoid damaging painted surfaces.

WHAT GERMS CAN HAND SANITIZER ELIMINATE?

Predictable, regular handwashing assists with eliminating germs and moderate the spread of microscopic organisms and infections that can cause colds and the flu. Unfortunately, it's not constantly conceivable to find a good pace with soap and water. Fortunately, on those occasions, it is frequently conceivable to spray some hand sanitizer gel that you can rub into your hands to keep them clean.

Scientists additionally note that the sorts of germs that hand sanitizers murder aren't the sorts that typically make you wiped out. While hand sanitizer may make your hands cleaner, it won't shield you from becoming ill. A few examinations, however, have indicated that standard hand sanitizer use can diminish the number of days people tend to fall sick.

As indicated by the 2014 survey, ethanol is incredible to such an extent that a couple of studies have discovered that in high focuses, it's better at disposing of three types of disease-causing microscopic organisms — Escherichia coli, Serratia marcescens, and Staphylococcus Saprophyticus — juxtaposed to washing hands with standard or antibacterial soap.

DOES HAND SANITIZER FAIL?

Alcohol is a rack stable synthetic as indicated by its security information sheet. This implies if alcohol is kept in a fixed compartment at room temperature, it will stay at a similar focus for an extremely long time.

Be that as it may, alcohol vanishes effectively on account of its generally low breaking point, and after some time, as the container is opened and shut, some alcohol may getaway, and the effectiveness of alcohol in your hand sanitizer may begin to diminish. All things considered, if you keep the container shut and at room temperature, you're probably going to have a successful item for as long, you need it.

SAFETY CONCERNS OF HAND SANITIZERS

There are certain safety concerns we should be aware of, especially when it comes to using sanitizers all the time.

Using hand sanitizers occasionally won't hurt, but regular use over time can actually lead to a number of safety concerns. In case you're wondering, here are some of them:

1. Dry Skin

The alcohol that's present in hand sanitizers can actually cause your skin to dry out. Since it's stripped away of natural oils, your skin will be more prone to irritation. Apart from that, it can also increase your risk of getting dermatitis.

2. Exposure to Toxic Chemicals

Hand sanitizers normally contain chemicals. However, if yours is scented, then it's likely that it contains a lot of toxic chemicals. The problem is that manufacturers aren't required to disclose which chemicals were used to create their products. As a result, you won't really have any idea which toxic chemicals you're exposed to when using such products.

One such example of these chemicals is parabens which are used for prolonging a product's shelf life. There's also phthalates which can disrupt your endocrine system, leading to a number of problems.

3. Accelerated Aging

Since hand sanitizers can cause your skin to dry out, it can also lead to the appearance of wrinkles and fine lines. As you keep on using sanitizers on a regular basis, its alcohol will disrupt your skin's natural barrier function. As a result, it will no longer be effective in protecting itself which, in turn, can lead to dehydration and eventually, accelerated aging.

4. Not that Effective

According to the FDA, there's no evidence to prove that hand sanitizers can be more effective than the old-fashioned handwashing using soap and warm water in order to prevent germs and viruses from spreading.

In fact, a study conducted in 2000 revealed that sanitizers don't actually reduce the amount of bacteria on your hands. Instead, they might even do the opposite which is increase the total bacterial count. They also added that since hand sanitizers can strip natural oils off your skin, using them on a regular basis can actually reduce your skin's layer of defenses.

WHICH IS MORE EFFECTIVE?

A hand sanitizer's effectiveness can actually depend on a number of factors, some of which include the duration of exposure, how it is applied, frequency of use, the quantity used, and whether the specific germs on your hands are vulnerable to the sanitizer's ingredients or not.

Generally speaking, alcohol-based sanitizers are capable of significantly reduce tons of bacteria, fungi, and even certain viruses as long as they're thoroughly rubbed on your hand for at least 30 seconds and paired with complete air drying. The same can also be true to their alcohol-free counterparts.

However, you have to keep in mind that sanitizers aren't capable of dealing with nonenveloped viruses as well as bacterial spores. Moreover, they aren't fully effective when applied to dirty or soiled hands.

Even though they can vary in terms of effectiveness, using hand sanitizers will allow you to regulate the transmission of infectious diseases. This is particularly essential in settings where handwashing is poor.

To conclude, alcohol-based sanitizers have been proven to be the more effective option. Just make sure to go for ones that have around 65-90% alcohol content, otherwise, it won't be that effective at all. However, even though alcohol-free versions aren't as effective as their alcohol-based counterparts, they're still effective solutions when it comes to killing germs on our hands.

BEST SANITIZER FOR YOUR SKIN TYPE

Sanitizers often differ in their main components, which have different effects with different types of skin. Due to that, it is essential to know what is the most compatible sanitizer to your skin to reap the best result. Here are the different type of sanitizer and their compatible skin types:

Chlorine Based

The sanitizers commonly sold to the public are chlorine-based. Chlorine is also referred to as bleach. It is useful in eliminating bacterias while still allowing consumers to stay within budget. However, its effectiveness is mitigated when the temperature level reaches the range of 55 F- 75 F.

This kind of sanitizer is perfect for normal skin types, as they are unlikely to develop adverse reactions. However, it is not ideal for those who have dry and sensitive skin. Bleach may cause dry skin type to be further dehydrated, resulting in flaking and irritation while it may cause chemical burns or rashes for sensitive skin types.

Quaternary Ammonia Based

When Quaternary Ammonia is diluted, it becomes non-toxic, colorless, and odorless, which makes it ideal for individuals with sensitive skin. This is because, among the other sanitizer compounds, this is the most gentle on the skin. It is also good for those who have oily and combination skin types.

The significant advantage of Quaternary Ammonia-based sanitizer is that it leaves an antimicrobial film layer once it is dry, which provides extended protection to the user. Moreover, unlike chlorine-based sanitizer, high temperature does not affect its effectiveness. However, its drawback is that it is slow-acting. It takes more time to kill bacterias compared to other types of sanitizer bases.

Iodine Based

Among all the sanitizer bases, this one is the fastest acting and most stable even in high temperatures. It is also effective against almost all kinds of bacteria, so it provides overall protection.

Iodine based sanitizers are commonly non-irritating to the skin. However, some skin types such as sensitive skins may develop chemical burn like rashes as a side effect. This is why, regardless of your skin type, it is best to use a patch test first to identify whether it is indeed compatible with your skin or not.

The primary purpose of sanitizers is to disinfect you from bacterias. However, they can also sometimes cause skin irritation if you are not careful.

This is why it is best to know your skin, read the labels, and test the product before investing in a big purchase.

2. DANGERS OF COMMERCIAL HAND SANITIZERS

First and foremost, let's talk about the use of commercially available hand sanitizers in children. It is tempting to use alcohol based sanitizers to decontaminate surfaces and some people use these products, not just on their hands but on the hands of their kids too. Even the CDC have reported the use of these alcoholic hand sanitizers in children and the risks it poses on their health. The most common adverse effects include irritation of the skin, eye problems or vomiting.

For these reasons, it is suggested to not use these hand sanitizers, particularly with kids 12 years or younger.

However, you do not need to worry. We have a solution for this problem provided in this very book. You will find recipes that contain all natural products that tend to have very few side effects, almost equal to none, and are less likely to cause irritation. We also have provided a special recipe of hand sanitizer that can be used particularly for children.

Another common problem that people face while using some (not all) commercial hand sanitizers is the use of triclosan. Let's discuss a bit about triclosan, what it actually is and why it is sometimes considered harmful.

Triclosan:

Triclosan is an antibacterial and antifungal chemical also called TCS. It is present in many common household products like toothpastes, soaps or detergents. Some companies use triclosan in their hand sanitizers too. Even though the use of triclosan in antiseptic washes was prohibited by FDA, it is still sometimes used in some products, and widely used in many other countries too. The ban by FDA in 2016 was due to the fact that there wasn't enough evidence to prove that it was safe to use. Still, the research regarding triclosan is inconclusive and it cannot be said with complete confidence that triclosan is as harmful as it is claimed to be. Many experiments have been conducted on mice to check the effect of triclosan. It was seen to cause inflammation in the gut and later studies have also provided evidence to show that it produces high levels of antibiotic resistant species in the gut.

Triclosan has been a subject of great controversy for a very long time. Even though considered as an antibacterial, the use of triclosan in topical medicines has been discouraged by many health care professionals. Some say that its excessive use can lead to alterations in immunity or cause hormonal problems. However, this is not confirmed yet.

To tackle this issue, it is important to look at the composition of hand sanitizers and see if they are triclosan based.

Many commercially available hand sanitizers contain thousands of chemicals in the name of fragrances. Since there is a great demand for nicely scented products, it is tempting to produce hand sanitizers that smell nice even if that means adding artificial products in it, some scented hand sanitizers can also cause massive irritation on sensitive skin. It can lead to respiratory problems, eczema and other associated issues that can prove to be dangerous with excessive use. Diseases like eczema and dermatitis can also be exacerbated with the use of these products.

We have a great variety of ways in which you can make hand sanitizers at home. In order to avoid the adverse effects of these commercially produced hand sanitizers, and to ensure good health, it is essential to know some homemade recipes too.

SAFETY CONCERNS

Alcohol is dangerous if ingested intentionally or not. Individuals seeking to abuse alcohol will likely ingest hand sanitizer. This could lead to death, poisoning, and the risk of fire. Alcohol is a highly flammable ingredient, producing a translucent blue flame. Some alcohol-based sanitizers may not produce this blue flame because of high concentrations of water and other moisturizing agents. Nevertheless, it's still flammable.

If a child is to use hand sanitizer, it should be used under the supervision of an adult. Other than that, it's necessary to keep it out of their reach. It shouldn't be rubbed around the eyes as it will cause inflammation. There should also be some restrictions placed on individuals (adults) who abuse or intend on abusing it to curtail access to these hand sanitizers.

WHO and Centers for Disease Control and Prevention (CDC) in the U.S promotes the culture of using alcohol-based sanitizers often, especially in work and school settings. They recommend using sanitizers that have at least 60% alcohol content. Most products that flaunt the market reportedly have between 60% and 90% alcohol. However, that doesn't mean they are more or less effective.

The use of some alcohol-free hand sanitizers hasn't really been in line with WHO and CDC's health vision. This is because these products do not offer maximum protection against infections. Concerns regarding the safety of the chemicals used in these alcohol-free hand sanitizers have often led the WHO and CDC to discredit their uses. Like the triclosan, for example, if this antimicrobial compound is used, it may interfere with the proper functioning of the endocrine system.

Hand sanitizers may no pose any threat to the skin, but they may strip the epidermis of oil, which will result in loss of skinlipid.

3. TYPES OF HAND SANITIZERS

What are the types of Hand Sanitizer?

Both types of hand sanitizer kills more or less harmful microorganisms. Compare your needs to your environment, budget, and personal preferences to choose the right product.

For example, if you work in a school, correctional facility, rehabilitation center, or manufacturing facility, an alcohol-free system will provide maximum safety and protection against swallowing and fire. If you work in a hospital that needs to follow strict FDA guidelines, you should use an alcohol-based gel. If you are seeming for a particular explication that you can carry in your handbag or backpack, you can also use gel. Alcohol-based tappers are frequently scantier and more contract than the foaming tools expected for non-alcoholic products. It is perfect for travel and mobile.

From a budget perspective, non-alcoholic hand sanitizers, which are often used per gallon, are cheaper. Each gallon costs the same, but typically uses 2,000 to 3,000 more foam disinfectants. This is because the dispensing mechanism of the solution adds air during use and advances the product further before it runs out. Regardless of your needs, use an effective hand sanitizer as part of a preventive defense against the disease.

ALCOHOL-BASED HAND SANITIZERS

The most common brands of disinfectants have alcohol as an active ingredient. The alcohol can be ethanol, isopropanol, or a mixture of the two compounds. Alcohol works by removing surface oils, including bacteria and viruses, from your hands. It further excludes most of these microorganisms by denaturing the proetids they receive. It also contains a moisturizer that prevents skin from drying out.

Mysteriously smooth subway poles, sneezing colleagues, the advent of the flu season: all of these are all reasons to thank bottles of alcohol-based hand sanitizers are within reach. The Age of Superbugs-Bacteria Resistant to Antibiotics-In the fear of not wanting to be clean, you may be wondering if constantly pouring puree into our palms would do more harm than harm. Recent studies have raised questions about the frequent use of alcohol-based hand sanitizers in hospitals. In a 2018 article written by Timothy, a researcher at the Doherty Institute and Immunity Institute at the University of Melbourne, the bacterium E. faecium has become more resistant " to alcohol-based hand sanitizers in hospital settings.

An environment that repeats the same actions over and over with the same chemicals, these bacteria and other microbes that can best survive under these conditions dominate this environment. "

But at the moment, this should not prevent the public from using the product, Larson said. "What we know now is that alcohol hand sanitizers are the fastest and best."

"The job of alcohol-based hand sanitizers is essentially to destroy bacterial cell walls," Larson says. Compared to water and soap, disinfectants are a convenient alternative on the go and are generally also more effective. "Alcohol is fairly powerful," Baron said, with the same 15-second wash with alcohol hand sanitizer compared to soap and water.

Alcohol as one of the
most commonly utilized disinfectants, liquor is known to have antibacterial properties. Solutions containing alcohols such as ethanol, isopropanol, and n-propanol are active antibacterial agents used as surgical spirits to disinfect the surface of the skin. Alcohol is effective against a wide range of bacteria and viruses because of its ability to denature and coagulate proteins. However, pure forms of alcohol are not as useful as antibacterial agents. This is because proteins do not denature appropriately without water. Therefore, an ideal alcohol solution, commonly known as cleaning alcohol, contains 60-95% alcohol.

Benefits and concerns of alcohol-based gel disinfectants

Alcohol-based products contain one of two active ingredients: alcohol or isopropanol. Both are effective preservative products that kill bacteria and bacteria. They share many of the same features. Their main difference is at the molecular level. A unique feature common to all of them is that they are highly flammable. Facilities must comply with local regulations and regulations when handling such flammable connections.

Another problem with alcohol-based hand sanitizers is the potential toxicity risk if swallowed. Most hand sanitizer dispensing mechanisms are easily opened. It will be placed in an accessible location to encourage use. Use caution when children and chemicals are in the same environment. Due to high alcohol concentrations, consumption by children and adults can lead to acute alcoholism.

A common side effect often associated with repeated use of alcohol-based hand sanitizers is dryness and cracks that can cause them in the hands. This is because alcohol removes oils from the skin that stores moisture. A temporary shortage of these oils may increase hand irritation to the surface. It can even cause dermatitis symptoms. Another complaint is that the alcohol in these products damages' floors and walls. Alcohol can contaminate areas where donors may drip or leak.

Alcohol-based products are the method (handwashing) recommended by major global health organizations such as CDC, WHO, and FDA. It is still the most commonly used disinfectant in hospitals and other medical facilities. Its effects have been proven over and over again.

ALCOHOL-FREE HAND SANITIZERS

Some organizations, such as B. Schools are concerned about the supply of alcohol-based products. Alcohol-free disinfectants are now available. These active ingredients are benzalkonium chloride, which has traditionally been used as a topical wound disinfectant. California researchers have tested the effectiveness of nonalcoholic disinfectants compared to elementary school handwashing and have found a significant reduction in children's illness.

The Pros and Cons of Alcohol-Free Hand Sanitizers:

Most non-alcoholic products available today are available in aqueous foam. The product contains the active ingredients benzalkonium chloride and quaternary ammonium. In contrast to alcohol-based products, alcohol-free hand sanitizers often contain less than 0.1% benzalkonium. They nevertheless implement the equivalent level of assurance. The rest of the solution is mainly composed of water and is often rich in skin care products such as vitamin E and green tea extract. It is non-flammable and relatively non-toxic due to its low benzalkonium concentration. However, all of these products are recommended for external use only.

Alcohol-free hand sanitizers have entered the market, addressing gel concerns and complaints. In many ways, they did it. In principle, these solutions are much easier for hands. Even if alcohol is accidentally ingested, the threat is much smaller, and alcohol-free hand sanitizers have a lower risk of fire and do not harm the surface. Another obvious advantage is extended protection. The ability of alcohol-based products to kill bacteria ends when the product dries on the skin. However, benzalkonium-based products provide protection even after the solution has dried. A possible disadvantage of alcohol-free solutions is that they are usually in the form of foam. This usually leads to a more comfortable experience for the user, but the dispenser requires a special foaming mechanism. This can significantly increase the cost of conversion from non-foamed systems because new hardware must be installed.

This is not to say that these organizations are not aware of the benefits of benzalkonium-based solutions. The term "non-alcoholic" can be applied to many products on the market. A spacious cycle that performs it impracticable for bureaus like the CDC and WHO to recommend it.

Alcohol- Based Hand Sanitizer Wipes

Antiseptic Wipes

Disinfecting wipes are generally effective for cleaning environmental surfaces, but are less effective for hands. Some products also contain alcohol. Disinfecting wipes with less than 40% alcohol are ineffective in this situation.

In the event of an emergency where soap, water, or hand sanitizers cannot be used, make sure that your sanitizing wipes contain at least 40% alcohol. Use caution when using disinfecting wipes, as they may propagate the bacteria, not remove them. Disinfecting wipes are intended for environmental cleaning and should be used only on the surface. The use of a damp cloth on multiple surfaces only pollutes the environment, not disinfect it. Therefore, disinfecting wipes are not a reliable option when dealing with new types of virus.

Due to the hardness of the product, disinfecting wipes should be used to clean the area, not the hands. Although, it is greatly suggested that you obtain an outcome that receives at least 40% alcohol.

Studies have shown that disinfecting wipes can sprinkle bacteria instead of actually killing them. Whenever possible, choose water and soap or a hand sanitizer instead.

Hand Sanitizer Sprays

Another form of hand disinfectant is spray. Alcohol-based disinfecting sprays are very beneficial.

And use it all over the world.

4. EFFECTIVENESS OF HAND SANITIZER

Hand sanitizers are proven to be very useful and effective, especially in the fight against viruses and infectious diseases. However, their effectiveness depends on the quantity used, frequency, and whether the disease-causing agents, pathogens, and infectious agents are likely to be affected by the active ingredients in the hand sanitizer.

Alcohol-based sanitizers, if rubbed thoroughly in-between the fingers, palms, and the back of the hands for about 30 - 45 seconds, followed by air-drying can reduce bacteria, certain types of viruses, and fungi to the barest minimum. Though it's less effective than alcohol-based sanitizers, alcohol-free sanitizers with BAC have similar effects in responding to bacteria and certain types of viruses.

Hand sanitizers can be used in nursing homes and hospitals exits, and in many public washrooms. We all know the importance of proper handwashing to reduce the insecure transmission of the germs. There are times, though, when there is no access to soap and water or insufficient time for thorough washing.

HOMEMADE SANITIZER ARE EFFECTIVE TO KILL GERMS

Waterless hand sanitizer provides some benefits over the soap and water hand cleaning.

Where organic matter (dirt, food, or other material) is visible on hands; they are not successful.

Some will also boost skin condition.

Anyone who has been in the play area of a child has experienced this. As the kids get off the play equipment, the mothers reach into their bag to get their hand sanitizer. The idea is this approach will keep the children safer, and their families.

- How much is it you can use?

Place a small volume, the size of your thumbnail, on the palm of your hand to use hand sanitizers efficiently, and rub it over your whole side, including your nailbeds. If the gel evaporates completely in under Fifteen seconds, you haven't used enough stuff.

- Limitations:

Not all hand sanitizer is produced equal. Look for active ingredients in the bottle. The quality of alcohol may be in the form of ethyl alcohol, ethanol, or isopropanol. Those are all suitable types of alcohol. Be sure that whatever form of alcohol is mentioned, its concentration varies between 60 and 95 percent. To be successful, the alcohol content of less than 60 percent is not enough.

• Doesn't cut alcohol by grime.

If the alcohol in the sanitizer must work, all dirt, blood, and soil must first be cleaned away or washed away.

Using hand sanitizers is a practice that can help keep all of us exposed to fewer germs and can thus reduce our risk of becoming sick. Whether you're on the playground, using someone else's machine, or visiting a hospital mate, take the time to rub a few on your fingertips. It represents a simple step towards a safe winter season. During the peak respiratory virus season [around November to April], the portable hand sanitizers do have a function as they make it much easier to clean your hand. It's much easier to wash your hands when you are sneezing than using a hand sanitizer, particularly when you're outdoors or in a vehicle. The hand sanitizers are much more convenient, and people are more likely to clean their hands, so this is better than not washing at all.

According to the Centers for Disease Control (CDC), it must be used correctly for hand sanitizer to be successful. That involves using the right amount (read the label to see how much you can use it), then rubbing it on all hand surfaces until your hands are warm. Should not dry your hands after applying or wash them. There is no evidence of dangerous hand sanitizers dependent on alcohol and other antimicrobial materials. Theoretically, they may contribute to antibacterial resistance. This is the most widely cited explanation of why people argue against using hand sanitizers. But that wasn't confirmed. No evidence of resistance to alcohol-based hand sanitizers has been identified at the hospital. While no studies are suggesting that hand sanitizers certainly pose a threat, there is also no proof that they are doing a better job of protecting you against harmful bacteria than soap. And even in hospitals or when you can't get to a sink, hand sanitizers have their place, washing with soap and warm water is almost always a better option.

HOMEMADE SANITIZER CAN BE YOUR TRAVEL CLEANING BUDDY.

Occasionally when you need it most, you can't find a commercial hand sanitizer in store. In some instances, washing your hands thoroughly in warm soapy water is more successful than using the hand sanitizer. Though, it isn't always easy to wash your hands with soap while you are traveling on flights or public transport. In this case, the hand sanitizer is a reasonable substitute. In travel size packets, you can take hand sanitizer into an airplane in your hand luggage.

Steps to Create DIY Hand Sanitizer Gel for Travel:

- Take two parts 91 percent rubbing alcohol (or stronger)
- Take 1-part aloe vera gel
- Mix in a cup
- Fill a travel squeezable bottle smaller than 3.4 oz or 100 ml

Steps to Create DIY Hand Sanitizer Shower for Travel:

- Take rubbing alcohol with a 75 percent minimum alcohol level
- Add 1.5 ml glycerol to 98.5 ml rubbing alcohol
- Mix in a bowl together.
- Use a fuel to fill a travel size pump spray bottle that is smaller than 3.4 oz or 100 ml
- Make sure the spray bottle has a cap to avoid unintended pump pressing

Know hand sanitizers are less effective when the hands are greasy, sticky, or dirty. Hand sanitizer isn't a replacement for soap and water to wash your hands when you get the opportunity. Many health experts aren't advocating making your sanitizer. This is mostly because they're afraid you'll end up with an unsuccessful drug. Even if you have a store-bought hand sanitizer, hand washing is a must. When you carry your homemade sanitizer onto a flight in your hand luggage, it would need to be in a container of travel size below 3.4 oz or

100 ml. Don't fill the bottle up to the top you need to clear some room for the liquid to expand or contract due to air pressure changes. Since hand sanitizer is a liquid, you do need to pack it inside your clear toiletries bag for quarter plastic. Some people prefer to use a pump-dispenser jar. If you want a bottle like this, then make sure it has a cap to avoid spilling the liquid when it's in your pocket, other people have used bottles like a roll-on deodorant with rolling ball dispenser.

Your best choice could be your old empty travel-size hand sanitizer bottle, so if empty, don't throw it away. You may have read that alcohol is banned on planes by more than 70% percentage. That still holds for alcoholic drinks. Without question, you can take rubbing alcohol, which is more durable than 70%. You can make your hand sanitizer that is as good as a hand sanitizer purchased from a pharmacy. Nonetheless, hand sanitizer alone might not be the only way to avoid picking up germs while at airports or riding in flights. A sanitizer product is just an instrument in your toolkit. You should undoubtedly have antibacterial wipes in your flight packing list too.

These can be used to clean off the tray table and armrest. Try waking up early and going on the day's first flight if necessary. Aircraft are typically washed and disinfected overnight; the first flight of the day is when the plane is mostly clean. When you are using a hand sanitizer, handwashing with soap and warm water is always necessary.

Wash your mouth, if you have the chance. Viruses are also spread by coughing and sneezing. It doesn't matter that how clean your hands are if you sit next to someone throwing a virus droplet out into the open.

5. BENEFITS OF YOUR HOMEMADE HAND SANITIZER

THE ADVANTAGES OF HOME-BASED INDUSTRY OF SANITIZERS

Home-based company shall be any company where the primary office is situated in the home of the owner. You don't need to buy the house, but you need to operate a business from the same premises that you live in to make the business home business. Though we expect home-based business owners to operate at home, this is not always the case. Computer engineers, truckers, and interior decorators are just three examples of people who may operate home-based businesses but must travel to provide their services.

There are several things while running a home business that attracts people to it, especially when it comes to spending and tax savings.

Private liberty: When you're used to wasting hours in traffic every day to and from work, two of the most exciting benefits of starting a home-based company are your newfound independence and the recovery of lost time. According to the US, the average American spends 348 hours of commuting per year. Suddenly, you have some extra hours with a home-based company to regain control of your personal life. Plus, there's no bosses, no dress code, no fixed schedule of work, and no maneuverable bureau politics. What you need is personal motivation, consistency, and the ability to manage time.

You get to keep the money that you are making. It is a basic principle: the harder you are working, the more money you can make. The potential of your earning is directly proportional to your results, so you don't need to wait for a promotion or a raise. You are working more and delivering better. You'll save gas and food money too. Home lunch planning is more cost-effective and provides a good break in the workday.

Gain potential: Starting your own home-based business with so many businesses and sectors in a recession means you can build your own income-producing opportunities.

In certain sectors, good job prospects can be scarce, and promotional incentives within major companies are also diminishing.

Danger less: Running a business from home requires even less cash for start-ups than a freestanding business or even a franchise. And once the company is up and running, managing it is cheaper and simpler than having a separate company place.

Tax incentives: There is a range of tax benefits of getting your home and office under one roof. As company expenses, you can subtract a portion of the operating and depreciation expenses of your house. It can be a percentage of your mortgage, income taxes, insurance, electricity, and/or household maintenance expenses.

Time for family and friends: This is particularly important for parents of school-age children: when they return, you will see the children off to school and be home on most days. Sometimes, if someone's sick, leaving the desk in your home is better than leaving one in the office of another.

Less exhaustion: Juggling the pressures of work and family is a little less difficult when you know you can stay home to care for a sick child and simply set your own timetable.

Professional development incentives: Having your own boss gives you the ability to wear loads of hats: sales director, marketing specialist, consultant, manager of business growth, and more. This gives you knowledge and experience in all aspects of running a company, which in effect makes you marketable even more.

Growing efficiency: Now that you no longer have to budget time and energy for commuting or a series of pointless meetings, you will have far more time and energy to make the success of your company.

An innovative springboard: Launching your home can be an opportunity for you to put your interests and hobbies into being and create a cash-generating platform for your unique and creative talents.

KEEP YOURSELF CLEAN USING RELIABLE SOURCES

Good skin pH is about 5.5 has higher pH in most traditional hand sanitizers—trusted Source, as 11. "If the pH of the skin is too high, the body will produce excess sebum to fight back and restore its normal pH. However, the residue from the sanitizers ensures that the destructive pH is preserved, "says independent beauty chemist David Pollack. "The end result is skin may get too oily. If that's not bad enough, the residue of the sanitizers emulsifies or attaches to the lipid matrix of the skin. "

But the advantage here is that if you're going to make your own sanitizer, then you're going to make it according to your needs, which will help you clean and keep you healthy.

6. IMPORTANCE OF HAND SANITIZATION

The usage of hand disinfectants is a part of the procedure for fantastic pollution control for employees working in hospital surroundings, or people involved with aseptic processing and inside cleanrooms. Even though there are lots of distinct sorts of hand sanitizers accessible that there are differences using their efficacy, and many don't match the European standard available sanitization.

Employees operating in hospitals and cleanrooms take various kinds of microorganisms in their palms, and these germs can be easily transferred from person to person or by individual to gear or surfaces that are critical. For critical surgeries, some security is given by sporting gloves. However, gloves aren't appropriate for many gloves and activities or even frequently sanitized or, if they're of an improper layout, can pick up and move contamination.

Hence, the sanitization of palms (either gloved or ungloved) is an equally significant part contamination management in hospitals, to steer clear of staff-to-patient cross-contamination or before undertaking surgical or clinical procedures; and also, for aseptic trainings such as the dispensing of medications. Additionally, not only is that the usage of a hand sanitizer required before undertaking these programs, it's likewise essential that the sanitizer is good at removing a large population of germs. Various studies have revealed that when a very low number of germs persist following the use of a sanitizer; subsequently, the subpopulation can grow, which can be resistant to potential programs.

There are lots of commercially available hand sanitizers having the most frequently used forms being alcohol-based fluids or dyes. Much like other varieties of disinfectants, hand sanitizers are effective against different germs based upon their style of action. Together with the most typical alcohol-based hand sanitizers, the manner of activity contributes to bacterial cell passing through cytoplasm leakage, denaturation of protein, and ultimate cell lysis (alcohols are among those so-called 'membrane disrupters'). The benefits of using alcohols as hand sanitizers incorporate a comparatively low price, small odor, and a fast evaporation (restricted residual activity contributes to shorter contact times). Additionally, alcohols have an established cleansing activity.

In picking a hands sanitizer, the pharmaceutical business or clinic will have to think about whether the program will be forced into human skin to gloved hands or to either, and if it's necessary to become sporicidal. Hand sanitizers fall into two different classes: alcohol established, which can be more prevalent, and also non-alcohol based. Such factors affect both upon price as well as the health and security of the employees utilizing the hand sanitizer because most generally accessible alcohol-based sanitizers may lead to excessive drying of the skin; and also a few non-alcohols established sanitizers may be irritating to skin. Alcohol hand sanitizers are intended to prevent irritation through owning sterile properties (color and odor-free) and components that manage skin protection and attention via re-fatting agents.

Alcohols have a lengthy history of usage as disinfectants as a result of inherent antiseptic properties from bacteria and some viruses. To succeed, some water must be blended with alcohol to apply effect against germs, together with the very best variety falling between 60 and 95 percent (most industrial hand sanitizers are approximately 70 percent). The most widely used alcohol-based hand sanitizers have been Isopropyl alcohol or some type of denatured ethanol (for instance, Industrial Methylated Spirits). The more prevalent non-alcohol established sanitizers include either chlorhexidine or hexachlorophene. Additives may also be contained in hand sanitizers so as to grow the anti-inflammatory properties.

Before entering a hospital guard or wash area, hands must be washed with soap and warm water for about twenty minutes. Handwashing eliminates around 99 percent of passing microorganisms. After that, if gloves are worn out or not, routine hygienic hand disinfection ought to take place to get rid of some succeeding transient flora and also to decrease the danger of the contamination originating out of properties that are resident.

The method of hands sanitization is of fantastic significance since the potency isn't only with all the alcohol.

In summary, hand sanitization is a significant process for employees to follow along with pharmaceutical and healthcare settings. Hand sanitization is just one of the chief procedures for preventing the spread of disease in pollution and hospitals inside pharmaceutical operations. This essential degree of control demands the usage of a successful hand sanitizer.

7. CHEMICAL INGREDIENTS IN HAND SANITIZER AND HOW THEY WORK TO KILL GERMS AND PREVENT INFECTION

To make hand sanitizers, you need two major ingredients; antimicrobial agent and an Emollient.

You can add as many other additives as you fancy but these two ingredients are what you really need to make your hand sanitizer at home.

Now, let's see how each ingredient contributes to the efficacy of your hand sanitizer:

Emollients: Emollients are common ingredients used in cosmetic making for lubricating, moisturizing and protecting the skin.

Because you're going to add antimicrobial agents to your hand sanitizer, it is important that you also add an emollient that would help to protect your skin from the dangers of the chemicals contained in the hand sanitizer.

The two major emollients use to make hand sanitizers are Aloe Vera gel and Glycerin.

Aloe Gera Gel is derived from the Aloe Vera plant, and it has great skin protection and moisturizing properties.

Aloe vera is also commonly used to fight skin infections and irritation, as it contains its own natural antimicrobial compounds.

You can choose to use Aloe Vera gel straight from the plant if you have one in your garden but if not; you can buy any organic Aloe Vera gel online or from stores around you.

Glycerin on the other hand, is a sugar alcohol. It is a clear, colorless liquid that is often derived from coconut oil, soybean or palm oil.

This odorless, sweet-tasting liquid is very popular in the skincare industry due to its super-hydrating qualities.

It works to moisturize and protect your skin just like Aloe Vera gel however; it doesn't contain any natural antimicrobial agents unlike Aloe Vera Gel.

If you can't find Aloe Vera gel or Glycerin around you easily, you can use Vitamin E, or Coconut oil- Coconut oil is equally good- just melt it and add it to your formulation.

Antimicrobial Agents: Antimicrobial agents are what will kill off and disrupt the growth and spread of viruses and bacteria that may have found their way to your hands.

Have you ever sprayed insecticide directly on an offending roach or termite, or have you ever seen salt being applied directly on the skin of an earthworm?

As soon as the salt touches the worm's body, it begins to wiggle vigorously, obviously in pains and discomfort, until it dies.

That is exactly how these alcohols work; when you add antimicrobial chemicals to your hands, it attacks the bacteria and viruses, causing them pain and discomfort and that way, they are unable to lay eggs or spread, and within seconds, they die off along with any eggs they might have laid.

There are alcohol-based and alcohol-free antimicrobial agents. The alcohol-based antimicrobial ingredients include Ethanol, the major ingredient in Vodka, Isopropyl Alcohol, or n-propanol, which is commonly known as rubbing alcohol.

The alcohol-free ones include Triclosan and Benzalkonium Chloride (BAC), which are commercial-grade ingredients. You don't need these ingredients when making hand sanitizers at home especially for Corona virus prevention as the World Health Organization (WHO) has advised that alcohol-based hand sanitizers have been found to be more effective against Corona Virus.

When adding alcohols to your formulations, make sure you use at least 60% alcohols. What this means is that for every 3 tablespoons of hand sanitizer, at least 2 tablespoons must be alcohols.

So, let's say you are making 3 tablespoons of hand sanitizer with just Aloe Vera gel and rubbing alcohol, you have to use 2 tablespoons of rubbing alcohol and only 1 tablespoon of Aloe Vera gel.

You can go over 60%, and maybe even do 2 ½ tablespoons of alcohol to ½ tablespoon of Aloe Vera gel but make sure you never do less than 60% otherwise, your hand sanitizer wouldn't be as effective, and that puts you at risk.

If you'll be adding more additives like Fragrance or Essential oils, make sure you always add enough alcohol to compensate for the dilution caused by the additives.

Fragrance: You may, or may not need fragrance but most people like to add fragrance to their formulations so as to mask the strong odor of the antimicrobial ingredients.

If you prefer to use fragrance, I'll advice you to stick with natural-based fragrance. You don't want to add anything harsh or toxic since you'll be using your sanitizer a lot.

Remember, anything you put on your skin can penetrate and get into your blood stream so you have to be picky with your ingredients.

Opt for essential oils as your fragrance. You can use strawberry, cinnamon, lemon, or lavender essential oil.

These essential oils smell really good without your skin exposing you to harm

Essential Oils: For extra moisturizing and skin protection, you can add essential oils.

However, essential oils known as Germ Destroyer Essential Oils are often used due to their bacteria killing abilities.

Germ destroyer essential oils like Tea tree essential oil, Clove essential oil, Eucalyptus essential oil, Geranium Essential Oil, and Peppermint essential oil can fight off bacteria, fungus, and viruses without the negative downsides of Alcohol and Triclosan.

If you are making hand sanitizers for kids or babies, this is the perfect ingredient to use however, if you are making something to guard against the spread of corona virus, you have to add alcohol.

Preservatives: Except you are making large batches for sale, you don't have to add preservatives to your homemade hand sanitizer.

As long as you sterilize your tools and bottles before using them, your hand sanitizer will hold up for a long time because on their own, they are able to fight off pathogens however, if you plan to sell them, you can add natural, non-toxic preservatives like Vitamin E oil, Rose Geranium Oil, or Citronella.

8. HOW TO PROPERLY DISINFECT MY HANDS?

There are lots of conditions where you could pick up germs such as bacteria or viruses. It is possible to soil your hands even though you're at the restroom or tub; once you alter dirty garments or nappies; following scratching or draining your nose while carrying your own meals when cooking meals; whereas washing veggies, red or white meat, poultry fish or products and so forth.

Your hands may get dirty once you handle crap or clean your property. Hands may get hay when you are seeing the hospital or whenever you are visiting a sick person. It is possible to muddy your palms once you fondle a furry friend or eliminate animal waste. You risk becoming infected once you cure a wound or a cutback.

Staff involved with blood diagnostic and testing labs must take care of tens of thousands of samples of semen, blood, sera, and other sampling components which contain microbes, toxins, corrosives, and other ingredients that were infectious.

In a workplace environment, you need to make sure that employees wash clean and wipe their hands thoroughly whenever that they use the bathroom or bathtub to decrease the dangers of transporting gastrointestinal ailments. Each time you clean your hands, make certain you're using a soap which works up a fantastic yank as plain rinsing may leave traces of germs on your palms.

For washing your own hands in an efficient fashion, initially, take your watch off or bands out of your wrist and palms. Open the faucet, which releases warm water and then wash your hands correctly. Scrub the soap from the palms before a lather is formed.

Scrub completely up into the forearm, scouring your palms and wrists for 15-20 minutes. Wash out the nails, too, especially beneath your nails. Thereafter clean your hands in conducting hot water. For wiping your palms use your private towel and also for drying use an air drier.

For many healthcare facilities, including hospitals, physicians, nurses, and food prep areas, the corporation must place up signals to notify staff and people how to wash their hands over every sink.

However, most hand sanitizers are ineffective against norovirus and bacterial spores. Using soaps have been reported to be more effective against them. They are also inefficient when you have soiled hands before application. In this case, for hand sanitizers to fully work, you must have washed your hands with soap and water to remove the soil before applying a hand sanitizer. Hand sanitizers do not thoroughly cleanse the skin. Hence, the need to do handwashing before using a hand sanitizer.

You should also note that frequent use of alcohol-based hand sanitizers can cause dry skin and irritation, except an emollient or a moisturizing agent, is added to the content. The use of these agents will substantially cause less skin dryness and irritation, and the tendency to have dermatitis.

Use these detailed handwashing directions to assist keep germs out of your department and also lower sick days. According to the Globe Health Organization, the entire handwashing process must take about 40 to 60 seconds.

Damp your hands initially.

You can utilize either cool or warm running water. A sink loaded with standing water could be contaminated.

Step 1: Use soap.

Don't cut corners on it; apply enough of it to cover all surfaces of your hands.

Step 2: Scrub hands with each other.

Develop a lather by massaging your palms with each other.

Step 3: Place your right palm over the rear of your left hand.

Intertwine your fingers and massage your hands back forth to obtain the soap on the back of your hand and also in between fingers, after that repeat with your left hand over your right-hand man.

Step 4: Scrub hands along with interlaced fingers.

Rub palms back and forth, obtaining the soap between your fingers.

Step 5: Place rear of finger in the opposing hand.

Revolve your hands together.

Step 6: Hold left thumb with right hand.

Revolve right-hand man to scrub your left thumb, then repeat with your left hand ordering your right thumb.

Step 7: Clean cleared out palm with fingertips of right hand. Rotate clasped fingertips within the palm of your cleared out hand, after that rehash with clasped fingertips on you're cleared out hand within the hand of your right hand.

Step 8: Rinse your hands.

Make certain to remove all soap from the rear of your hands, hands as well as between your fingers.

Step 9: Dry hands.

Dry your hands thoroughly with a single-use paper towel.

Step 10: Turn off the tap.

Utilize the paper towel to turn off the tap.

Step 11: You are done.

Your hands are currently clean.

When to Clean Your Hands.

Constant hand-washing is just one of the best ways to stay clear of getting ill and also spreading out illness. The CDC recommends cleaning hands when they are noticeably dirty, or:.

Before:.

Preparing or eating food.

Treating injuries or taking care of a sick person.

Putting or removing call lenses.

After:.

Preparing or consuming food.

Using the bathroom or transforming a diaper.

Blowing your nose, coughing or sneezing.

Dealing with wounds or caring for a sick person.

Handling rubbish.

If soap and also water aren't readily available, you can make use of hand sanitizers instead. It needs to be an alcohol-based hand sanitizer that is at least 60% alcohol. Apply the product to one hand as well as scrub your hands with each other. Continue to scrub your hands and also fingers until all surface areas are covered and also your hands are completely dry.

When to Wash

. Always clean your hands after you utilize the bathroom, prior to you consume food, and also at any time your hands are noticeably dirty, states Janet Haas, Ph.D., R.N., supervisor of public health at Lenox Hill Healthcare Facility in New York and a head of state of the Organization for Professionals in Infection Control as well as Public Health. It's very easy to pick up or transfer bacteria in all 3 of these instances.

" People must additionally take into consideration cleansing their hands after they've gotten on public transport," she includes.

You ought to also clean your hands after dealing with raw meat, such as turkey or poultry.

Make sure children wash their hands when they come into your home after playing outside. The Centers for Illness Control and also Prevention likewise advises that you clean your hands after touching animals.

If you have a respiratory system infection, such as the cold or the influenza, you may intend to clean your hands more often than usual, Haas states. That's since if you're coughing and sneezing, you could be contaminating your hands as well as spreading the insect to others.

Be Specifically Careful at the Hospital.

Though hand health is always crucial, it's important if you remain in the hospital, where serious as well as in some cases antibiotic-resistant infections can prowl.

And while healthcare facility personnel ought to likewise be cleansing their hands faithfully, either by cleaning with soap as well as water or utilizing hand sanitizer, study shows that does not always take place. According to the CDC and also diverse researches, some service providers clean their hands as little as fifty percent as often as they should.

If you are hospitalized or looking after a person that is, and also notification that a healthcare provider hasn't depleted or made use of hand sanitizer when entering your space, speak out, by pleasantly asking whether he has washed his hands.

In addition, remind visitors to clean their hands when they go into as well as leave the area. As well as if you're the client, be sure to keep up with your hand hygiene. Ask for assistance cleaning your hands prior to a dish, or demand a container of alcohol-based hand sanitizer.

The Most Effective Means to Wash

. Normally, washing with soap and also water is one of the most reliable method for lowering the number of bacteria on your hands.

Plain soap is best. Avoid anti-bacterial products because there's no proof that they function any much better than normal soap, and also they may urge the breeding of bacteria that can't be healed by prescription antibiotics.

Scrub for 20 seconds, ensuring to wash the backs of your hands, between fingers, as well as under fingernails.

If you have no accessibility to soap and water, using a hand sanitizer made with at the very least 60 percent alcohol is the next best alternative. But hand sanitizers do not work as well when your hands are noticeably filthy, as well as they won't eliminate all type of germs.

For example, the CDC states as efficient as hand washing versus the highly transmittable stomach bug norovirus.

Properly to Wash Your Hands.

Another crucial kind of microorganisms are inadequate against is Clostridioides difficile (C. diff), which creates a hard-to-cure diarrheal infection that prevails in medical facilities. Hand sanitizers are thought about enough for some of the routine cleaning that medical care employees do sometimes a day, if you have C. diff, they (as well as you and any kind of site visitors) have to wash with soap and also water to stay clear of spreading out the infection.

ADVANTAGES OF PROPER HAND WASHING

Knowing the positive effect of handwashing on your life and family, for the most part, is a decent persuading component to stay aware of good clean propensities. The following are the most significant advantages of handwashing you should observe:

• Creating a more secure workplace for clinical staff and the patients

The idea of numerous sorts of clinical strategies is extremely sensitive. It, for the most part, manages uncovered inside organs or passing medications into the body. So in these specific cases, handwashing must be paid attention to because hurtful microbes can undoubtedly get into our bodies to cause more damage. Great clinical offices have fundamental facilities for effectively available handwashing. These facilities ought to be utilized routinely by specialists, patients, and guests.

Also, those offices should be completely sterile, and soap containers, sanitizers, and different things should be recharged routinely. Likewise, exceptional waste removal units should be in the washroom, too.

The efforts for making a more secure workplace additionally incorporate a more exhaustive and more point by point hand cleaning than it is normal from different representatives. There is a sure way personal clinical plans for the medical procedures and intercessions, and it requires a great deal of top-notch soap.

• Prevention of looseness of the bowels and uncomfortable intestinal diseases

Contact with fecal issues weighed down with the causative microscopic organisms can prompt the looseness of the bowels and intestinal diseases. Ordinary washing of the hands will evacuate this fecal issue and microbes from our hands in any event, when we have reached them from others or items.

The new microbes that an individual acquaints with their intestinal framework by filthy hands wreck the equalization, which is hard to reestablish.

• Avoidance of normal eye diseases

Eye contaminations are normally brought about by the microscopic organisms that get into the eyes from our hands. Hopefully, you will cease from contacting your eyes with your exposed hands. Be that as it may, as a rule, it happens automatically.

Therefore, it is ideal for handling this in another manner. Control what you can – wash your hands. Keeping the hands clean by customary washing will forestall regular contaminations.

In any case, the basic eye diseases that occur because of direct contact with various germs are:

Conjunctivitis (pink eye)

Keratitis

• Obstruction of respiratory tract contaminations

Similarly, the germs that cause these contaminations are generally found on grimy hands. Ordinary washing of the hands will expel these germs effectively, guarding you.

Germs that cause respiratory contaminations to incorporate microbes, infections, and even a few organisms. The indications can be very basic for every one of them:

• Coughing
• Sneezing
• Runny nose
• Nasal release
• Nasal clog

Most instances of flu are brought about by infections being transmitted to the wet patches of the face by messy hands.

• Reduction of the microbes content on your hands

Microbes have been known to wait on the hands and different items for days! This implies if you don't wash your hands anticipating that the microbes should bite the dust, you may be in for a shock. They will remain on your hands, or surprisingly more terrible, advancing toward your eyes or mouth, causing contaminations.

Remember to pay additional care to wash underneath part of your nails. Those that are inclined to nail chewing may experience the ill effects of numerous upsetting results.

• Keeping your work environment liberated from microscopic organisms

Ordinary cleaning of ordinarily utilized office gear with an alcohol-based cleaning item can lessen the number of microorganisms on them.

In any case, this doesn't spare you from their essence. You ought to likewise wash your hand routinely to keep your hands from being the medium through which the microorganisms that are hauled all around the workplace.

9. WORLD HEALTH ORGANIZATION (WHO) - RECIPE FOR CREATING ALCOHOL BASED HAND RUB

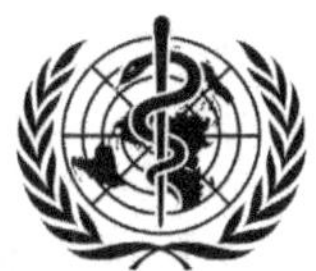

How to make a home-made hand sanitizer according to World Health Organization (WHO)

A The WHO produced a document (WHO, 2020) showing the directions to follow when making a hand sanitizer. Here are the tips to follow.

The Ingredients

2.2 gallons of ethanol 96% or 2 gallons of Isopropyl alcohol 99%.

Hydrogen Peroxide 3%. This chemical kills bacterial spores that may contaminate the hand sanitizer. You require 1.76 cups, which is similar to 471 ml.

Glycerol 98%. It acts as a moisturizer and amounts to 145ml.

Sterile distilled water or cold boiled water.

Materials needed to mix the ingredients

Depending on the amount of hand sanitizer you want to make, you may need a plastic container with a volume of 2.6 gallons to as much as a 50-liter tank.

Plastic or wooden spoons for mixing.

Measuring jug and measuring cylinder.

Plastic funnel.

An alcoholmeter.

Directions

This recipe provided by the World Health Organization can be made in a 10-liter glass container.

Here is a step by step preparation:

The alcohol is added into the container until the graduated mark.

Hydrogen peroxide is added after measuring the correct amount.

Place glycerol into the mixture.

The sterile distilled water is then used to top up the mixture to the 10-liter mark.

A lid is capped onto the container as soon as you add the water to prevent evaporation

The solution is mixed gently.

Keep the solution unopened until after 3 days. This period allows for bacteria and viruses in the alcohol to get destroyed.

You can then transfer the resulting solution into small squirting bottles that can be carried easily wherever you go.

For a bigger cluster of hand sanitizer, the World Health Organization (WHO)Trusted Source has a formula for a hand sanitizer that employs:

isopropyl alcohol or ethanol

hydrogen peroxide

glycerol

bubbled cold water

CONSTITUTION OF ALCOHOL-BASED FORMULATIONS FOR IN-HOUSE/NEIGHBORHOOD CREATION.

The selection of segments for WHO handrubs considers both cost imperatives and microbiological viability. The obtainment of crude ingredients will be influenced by the accessibility of inadequate materials available, and it is essential to choose nearby sources with care.

The accompanying two alcohol-based handrub formulations are prescribed for arrangement in-house or in a nearby creation office, up to a limit of 50 liters:

Formulation 1

To deliver ultimate concentration of ethanol 80% v/v, glycerol 1.45% v/v, hydrogen peroxide ($H2O2$) 0.125% v/v.

Formulation 2

To deliver ultimate concentration of isopropyl alcohol 75% v/v, glycerol 1.45% v/v, hydrogen peroxide (H_2O_2) 0.125% v/v:

CRUDE MATERIALS

While alcohol is the dynamic segment in the formulations, certain parts of different segments ought to be regarded. Every single crude material utilized ought to be ideally liberated from feasible bacterial spores. The crude materials for incorporation/thought are recorded underneath:

H_2O_2 Hydrogen Peroxide:

• The low convergence of H_2O_2 is expected to help kill tainting spores in the mass arrangements and isn't a functioning substance for hand antisepsis.

• H_2O_2 includes a significant wellbeing perspective, anyway the utilization of 3–6% for the creation may be confounded by its destructive nature and by troublesome acquisition in certain nations.

Glycerol:

• Glycerol is added as a humectant to build the worthiness of the item.

• Other emollients might be utilized for healthy skin, given that they are affordable, accessible locally, miscible (mixable) in water and alcohol, non-harmful, and hypoallergenic.

• Glycerol has been picked because it is protected and generally economical. Bringing down the level of glycerol might be considered to additionally diminish the tenacity of the handrub.

Utilization Of Acceptable Water

While sterile refined water is favored for making the formulations, bubbled and cooled faucet water may likewise be utilized as long as it is liberated from noticeable particles.

Utilization of different added substances (Additives)

It is firmly suggested that no ingredients other than those predetermined here can be added to the formulations.

In the instance of any extra additives, justification must be furnished together with reported wellbeing of the added substance, its similarity with different constituents, and every single important detail ought to be given on the item name.

Scents

The addition of scent isn't suggested in light of the danger of unfavorably susceptible responses.

Suggested measures of Products:

Isopropyl alcohol 99.8%: 7515 ml

Hydrogen peroxide 3%: 417 ml

Glycerol 98%: 145 ml

STEP BY STEP PROCEDURES

The alcohol for the formula to be utilized is filled in the tank to the graduated imprint.

Hydrogen peroxide is included utilizing the estimating chamber.

Glycerol is included utilizing an estimating chamber. As glycerol is exceptionally adhering to the mass of the estimating chamber, it ought to be washed with some sterile refined or cold bubbled water and then discharged into the jug/tank.

The bottle/tank is then bested up to the 10-liter imprint with sterile refined or cold bubbled water.

The solution is blended by shaking delicately were proper or by utilizing an oar.

FORMATION AND STORING

At whatever point conceivable and as indicated by nearby approaches, governments ought to energize neighborhood creation, bolster the quality appraisal procedure, and keep creation costs as low as could be expected under the circumstances. Unique prerequisites apply for the creation and amassing of the formulations, just as for the capacity of the crude materials. Since undiluted ethanol is exceptionally combustible and may light at temperatures as low as 10°C.

SECURITY STANDARDS

As to skin responses, hand-rubbing with alcohol-based arrangements is preferable endured over handwashing with soap and water. In an ongoing report led among ICU health-care workers, the momentary skin averageness and adequacy of WHO-suggested handrub formulations were essentially higher than those of a reference item. Any added substance ought to be as non-poisonous as conceivable if there should arise an occurrence of coincidental or deliberate ingestion.

74

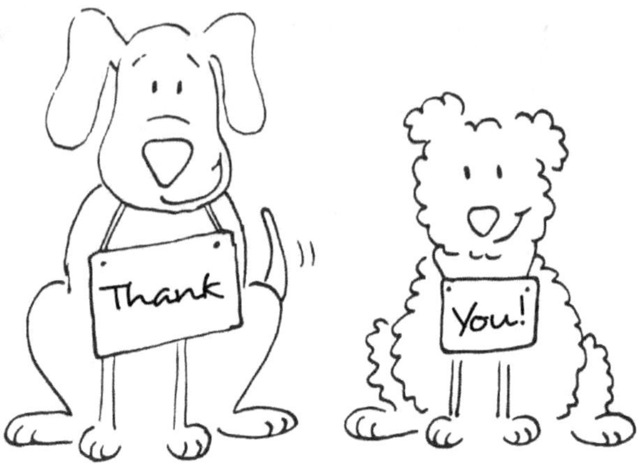

Enjoying this book so far?

I'd love it for you to share your thoughts and post a quick

review on Amazon!

10. MYTHS AND MISCONCEPTIONS ABOUT HAND SANITIZERS

There are various misconceptions and myths regarding hand sanitizers. Within this guide, we are going to have a look at a few details to debunk the myths and put the record right.

Among the most well-known misconceptions is that hand sanitizers are almost infallible, and they can stop the spread of contagious diseases, for instance, cold or influenza. Even though a hand sanitizer may kill over 60% of influenza viruses onto your hands, many people really contract influenza from airborne representatives, by breathing at the germs. Thus, even in the event that you've employed a sterile merchandise, and your hands are fresh and germ-free, you're still able to catch or spread the virus. A hand sanitizer might actually be much stronger preventative mechanism for gastrointestinal ailments, instead of illnesses like the flu or cold.

The other myth is they are much less effective as traditional handwashing with soap and water, also in eliminating germs in your hands on. This isn't always correct. Washing with water and soap functions betters in case your hands are obviously soiled, in other words, in case you've got dirt from your hands. But in case your hands look fresh but are now intercepted using germs; subsequently, an alcohol-based hand sanitizer is still a better choice since the alcohol is significantly more successful in eliminating the germs.

The next myth is that hand sanitizers cause dry hands. These products include emollients that are compounds that reduce aggravation by soothing and protecting skin. As counterintuitive as it might look, an alcohol-based hand sanitizer is really less harsh on skin than soap and water. A research conducted by Brown University researchers found that washing your hands with water and soap contributes to skin, which may appear and feel very dry. A hand sanitizer on the opposite hand can keep hands sterile.

You're able to earn a somewhat powerful sanitizer in the home. While homemade versions might be more economical, most do not include the recommended 60 percent alcohol content, which experts agree is that the best concentration to get rid of germs. The best results are observed with new names, for example, Purell or even Germ X.

However, provided that the item includes 60% alcohol, some generic manufacturer may work just as good as a superior store brand new. You do not need to pay the high cost for a brand name merchandise.

Compiling all of the hand sanitizer truth, we may safely state an alcohol-based sanitizer has become easily the best ways to kill germs from our own hands but just provided that the item is used properly and efficiently.

Alcohol-based sanitizer isn't just able to remove more germs than water and soap, but it's also gentler in skin when used in moderate quantities. When supervised by an adult, this item could be safe for children too.

While alcohol-based sanitizers have confronted criticism of late, but largely as a result of alcohol concentration, specialists say that a few of those fears are unfounded. Alcohol isn't absorbed into skin into some level to justify these anxieties. In spite of excessive utilization, the degree of alcohol consumption is benign in the top. Alcohol can contribute to a sanitizer risks, but not to any wonderful extent.

The debate against alcohol material only holds up when the goods are employed in a manner, they weren't meant to be utilized in. By way of instance, an alcohol-based hand sanitizer isn't supposed to be consumed; however, there have been a number of instances where children in addition to adults have swallowed the liquid and dropped very sick.

Some producers have tried to deal with the public's concern over alcohol material and began producing alcohol-free versions as a safer choice. These products rely upon plant oils neutralize germs, but to date haven't been as successful as alcohol-based hand sanitizers. If utilized correctly, an alcohol-based hand sanitizer isn't any more harmful than an alcoholic free version.

Risks in making your own hand sanitizer

Is ethanol the best alcohol to use?

First and foremost, what is an ethanol? Well, an ethanol is also known as alcohol, grain alcohol, and ethyl alcohol, which is a vivid and colorless liquid. Due to the fact that it can eagerly dissolve in many organic compounds including water, it is also an ingredient in many products produced, beginning from paints and varnishes to fuel to personal care and beauty products.

It is also a common ingredient in various beauty products and cosmetics and it works as an astringent to assist neat skin, in lotions as a preservative and also to support to make sure that the ingredients in the lotion do not move in different directions.

As a result of the fact that it is effective in eliminating microorganisms like fungi, viruses, and bacteria, it is presently an ingredient that is common in various homemade sanitizers. In America, the Centers for Disease Control and Prevention (CDC) recommends people to make use of homemade sanitizers in places where both water and soap are unavailable.

It should be noted that it is highly flammable and one shouldn't make use of it close to open flames. Also, its inhalation can lead to you coughing or having headaches too, although it has been labelled by the FDA that is safe to use in any food product. Why is this so? This is due to the fact that it comes fully from alcohol.

Alcohol that is safe for the skin Products specifically for the skin are so sophisticated, with list of ingredients that are usually difficult to pronounce or very long. In terms of alcohol, it is usually perceived as unsafe for the skin, but it is also part of the ingredient that should be researched on Well, to cut the long story short, we are actually going to give in details whether alcohol is good for the skin or not.

With the fact that various individuals have imagined that every alcohol product are unsafe for the skin, well, this is far from the truth if you must know. There are various distinctive types of alcohols, with distinctive uses and distinctive health impacts. A few are considered to be safe when they are used, while some others are unsafe.

In addition to this, there are a few initial red flags to assist you know if your product, that is, homemade sanitizer, possesses a good or bad alcohol content. Assuming that you select a hand sanitizer and discover that the main ingredient is an alcohol, it is fair enough to say this is a bad product, and you might want to do thorough research before buying the product from your location.

Back to what we were discussing, it should be noted that fatty alcohols are derived from coconuts or nuts, which both of them are natural ingredients. These types of alcohols add cetyl alcohol which is originated from stearyl alcohol and coconut oil. Also, these alcohols are used mainly as emulsifiers; to assist get a luxurious and firm texture in hand sanitizers or any skin care product.

As a result of the high content the fatty acids possess, these types of alcohols have a good

Effect on your skin. It also possesses emollient properties, indicating they assist to increase your skin's defensive barrier by either safeguarding your skin from damage or locking in moisture.

Generally, fatty alcohols are considered safe, thus, when you buy any skin care product or any hand sanitizer and you see stearly alcohol or cetyl alcohol, do not be scared.

Finally, it should be noted among individuals that when making use of any alcohol product, ensure that it is just a rinse-away product, such as cleansers. You should not use alcohols in products such as primers, serums, or even creams.

Alcohol that is unsafe for the skin the alcohols that are not safe for the skin are either denatured alcohols or simple alcohols, which are designed with the use of petroleum-based ingredients. In another meaning, it is something that one would not like to use on his or her skin or even bloodstream. These types of alcohols do not include isopropyl alcohol, ethanol, and alcohol denat. Many of them are often used as preservatives, while a few others are used as skin care formulas to the perfect textures, and also some are used to assist liquid formulas, and finally some of them are added in toners and cleaners to assist limit too much sebum.

Although, it might come with its benefit by having short-term impacts for people suffering from acne and also people with oily complexions, but they tend to dry your skin on the long run. When this type of alcohol is used regularly on a daily basis, it tends to weaken your skin's natural barrier by making the skin to be more difficult to retain elasticity and moisture.

It should be noted that these types of alcohol, when used regularly on a daily basis, can result to death, which can increase signs of aging like wrinkles and fine lines.

These alcohols, when used on a regular basis, are also not likely to have an overall effect on your body.

Finally, these alcohols may have the ability of causing skin irritation, breakouts, and wrinkles, although they are highly unlikely to pose a more severe hazard.

11.   WHAT TO DO WHEN HAND SANITIZER IS UNAVAILABLE

Normally, we are able to enjoy the luxury of going to the store to buy hand sanitizer when we need it. There are plenty of brands to choose from that offer a wide variety of benefits while also promising a pleasant scent or moisturizing properties.

What happens when the stores run out, though? When everyone is rushing to the stores to purchase the same products, the stores are bound to run out of them, and restocking doesn't happen fast enough to keep up with the demand.

Instead of panicking that you will have to go without hand sanitizer, you need to act wisely and avoid bulk-buying. When people purchase too much of a specific product during a time of extreme need, they put an undue stress on that product's production line and supply chain. Because stores can only supply individuals with so much of a certain product, you are actually putting others at risk by purchasing more than you need. While it is important to keep yourself and your family protected, understand that there are other ways you can do so; by using ingredients that you likely already have at home, you can make your own hand sanitizer.

It's also important to not underestimate the power of humble soap.

Because cleaning your hands with hand sanitizer is often easier than taking the time to wash your hands, you might have developed a preference for this method. To get your hands truly clean, you always need to wash them properly in a sink. Soap is going to kill more germs than hand sanitizer, so whenever it is possible, wash your hands this way. The convenience of hand sanitizer is only going to protect you when you combine it with a rigorous and regular hand-washing routine. As mentioned, if your hands become too used to one method, it isn't going to be as effective at killing all of the germs.

When you feel that you need to clean your hands, also remember to clean surfaces that you touch regularly. Using disinfecting wipes on your countertops, doorknobs, and other household surfaces will give you some peace of mind in knowing that you are doing your best to keep healthy. Don't forget about your car: your steering wheel can harbor a lot of germs and bacteria. Think about anything that you touch frequently, and do your best to sanitize it. Before you reach a state of panic, you must remember to think smart. Use the resources that you do have and get creative when you must.

Things to Remember

You should have your home equipped with necessary hygienic resources at all times. It is not a bad thing to make sure that your medicine cabinets are always stocked, and that your cleaning supplies are replenished often. These products provide you with several ways to stay healthy, so they should always be kept stocked up in your home as a priority. There is no need for a mass-purchase of these products, either. Keep a rational amount that makes sense for the number of people in your household.

Make up an emergency kit that can serve you in a time of need, for example during a natural disaster or a health crisis. In this kit, you should make sure to include proper bandages and wound-disinfectants. Provide yourself with plenty of ways to sanitize injuries, because this will give you a better chance of healing properly without developing infections. Include some space blankets and other ways that you can keep warm, because you never know what might happen with your utilities in an emergency situation. You might also have to take your kit to go, so make sure it's portable. Clean bottles of water that you regularly replace are also essential to keep in your emergency kit.

If anyone in your household needs to take prescription medication, be sure to include some in the kit. Any preventative medication (Advil, Tylenol, Ibuprofen, etc...) can also be included. Pack a thermometer, and make sure that you also pack some extra batteries. In case you do not have access to digital funds, it is important to also store some cash in the kit. As far as non-medical items go, be sure that each person has a pair of shoes and a basic change of clothes. For any pets that you have, be sure to add additional water and some dry or canned food. Do your best to make sure that everything is compact enough to fit in a single bag that you can store near an exit in case you must grab it and go quickly.

A bottle of rubbing alcohol or hydrogen peroxide is also essential, because this can sterilize different types of items and will be useful in case you do not have access to hand sanitizer or a sink. With any products that include an expiration date, make sure that you regularly check and replace them to ensure that your kit is up to date. When you can prepare for a difficult time this way, you won't be filled with so much panic in case of emergency. Having all of the supplies that you need in one place can offer you some peace of mind when you are in a situation that is unpredictable.

12.   SAFETY CONSIDERATION

Leading a healthy life is and should be the top most priority for every person. Being on a sick bed makes us realize how lucky being healthy is, and how grateful we should be for every moment we spend disease free.

The world that we are living in today is becoming increasingly dangerous. The reason is not just the political turmoil that every country is in, but also the increasing rate of natural calamities that we are facing.

With the start of the year 2020, we saw the world changing before our very eyes. Climate change was the real threat following us for the last few years, the fear of losing our planet to increasingly hazardous effects of carbon emissions.

HOW TO PREVENT YOURSELF FROM GETTING SICK:

Keep your hands clean

Wash, wash and wash

This has been our mantra from the very start. No matter what else you do to keep yourself safe from disease, do not forget that handwashing should be your number one priority. Handwashing alone can help save you from many illnesses.

Our hands consciously and unconsciously get in contact with many contaminated surfaces throughout the day, and when these hands touch the mucus membranes of the body, bacteria get a free pass inside you.

If you do not have access to clean water and soap everywhere, an alcohol based hand sanitizer can be your next best friend. Check out our recipes for homemade alcohol based hand sanitizers if you haven't already.

Eat green vegetables

A lot of people don't like eating vegetables, especially the boring greens. Well, this time you should keep in mind that the green vegetables are full of nutritious juices and a wide variety of vitamins. Taking plenty of vitamins can help keep you away from many diseases. It fortifies your immune system and helps you in fighting viral infections specifically.

Get proper sleep

We cannot stress more on how important sleep is to keep your body healthy and fit. Sleep essentially restores your body and makes you a new person every morning you wake up. Sleep replenishes your body and reinvigorates it. Another important thing to keep in mind is that an adequate amount of sleep helps you in fighting off microbes and helps in building resistance against viral attacks.

Get vaccinated!

Remember that the only thing that is going to save you from many fatal diseases is a dose of vaccine. Vaccine does not damage your body, and no, it does not give you more diseases. In simple words, it is merely a harmless form of microbes that is injected into your body so that the body can recognize it and build immunity. So, the next time that microbe attacks, your body will already know how to fight against it and will not be taken by surprise.

Take proper nutrition

Your body is going to build from the food you eat. If you eat healthy, your mind and body stays healthy, and if you don't, you get sick. There are many foods that can specifically help in building your immunity. We have made a list of a few foods to get you started:

Citrus fruits: Citrus fruits contain a large amount of vitamin C. Vitamin C is our saviour in fighting against diseases, specifically viral illness. It helps in building your immunity by increasing the number of white blood cells in the body. These include lemons, oranges, grapefruit.

Spinach: Ever wondered why the health experts always advise you to eat green veggies like spinach regularly? It is because spinach is a wonderous vegetable. It is not only rich in vitamin C but also provides your body with a wide variety of antioxidants to keep you healthy

Sunflower seeds: Not widely eaten, but sunflower seeds are packed with nutrients. The most important nutrient in these seeds is Vitamin E. Like vitamin C, vitamin E also helps to some extent in building your immunity. Vitamin E also acts as an antioxidant.

Now that we have briefly discussed how some important safety measures can help you stay away from diseases, let's get back to hand hygiene as it is the single most important factor in prevention of illnesses.

Hand sanitizers play a very important part in maintenance of hygiene. Water and soap are not accessible everywhere and that is why hand sanitizers can help ward off bacteria for some time. Like every other product, the efficacy of hand sanitizers also depend on its adequate usage. It is very important to know how to properly use these products and what safety concerns should be kept in mind while using them

We have already discussed the dangers posed by commercially produced hand sanitizers in. Here we will give you a quick summary on what to avoid and keep in mind while using hand sanitizers, whether commercially produced or handmade.

What to keep in mind while using hand sanitizers:

Hand sanitizers, while being very important for hygiene, do not substitute hand washing. These cannot be used on your hands if there is visible dirt on it. In these cases, you must wash your hands first to remove the dirt.

It is important to know the composition of the products that you are using. Products that contain large quantities of chemicals will do more harm than good.

Make sure that you are not using a large quantity of essential oils in your homemade preparations. Although essential oils give a soothing effect to the skin, excessive use is not advised.

Try to test a small quantity of whichever product you use on a small patch of skin first. Every person's skin is different and while one product is suitable for one skin, it might not be good for another person. In people that have sensitive skin type, using harsh chemicals or excessive drying of skin produces adverse reactions and may cause damage. It is important to report to a healthcare professional if you are having any serious symptoms

Keep these products out of the reach of children as many of them might contain ingredients that can be toxic if ingested orally. When you make hand sanitizers at home and do not label them or keep them away from the kids, there is a chance of accidental ingestion that might prove hazardous. In case it does happen, it is advisable to take the child directly to the emergency room and inform them timely.

In this book, we managed to educate you not only about the basics of hand sanitizer usage but also on the pros and cons and safety measures to take while using them. The wide variety of recipes, can help in saving you from all the trouble and help you in making hand sanitizers at home. Remember, prevention is better than cure and together we can fight against any calamities that may befall.

13. DISPARITIES BETWEEN HAND SANITIZER, HAND SOAP AND WATER

WHEN WOULD IT BE A GOOD IDEA FOR ME TO UTILIZE HAND SANITIZER?

Alcohol-Based Hand Sanitizer

Before and after visiting a companion or a friend or family member in a medical clinic or nursing home, except if the individual is debilitated with Clostridium Difficile.

• If soap and water are not accessible, utilize an alcohol-based hand sanitizer that contains at any rate 60% alcohol, and wash with soap and water when you can.

When would it be a good idea for me to utilize Soap and water?

Before, during, and in the wake of planning nourishment

Before taking nourishment

Before and in the wake of thinking about visiting somebody that is ill.

Before and in the wake of treating a cut or wound

After utilizing the washroom, evolving diapers, or tidying up a youngster who has utilized the restroom

After blowing your nose, coughing, or wheezing

After contacting a creature,

After contacting trash

If your hands are unmistakably grimy or oily

By what means would it be a good idea for me to utilize a Hand Sanitizer?

Use an alcohol-based hand sanitizer that contains at any rate 60% alcohol. A few circumstances where utilization of a hand sanitizer might be suitable to incorporate when you're riding open transportation, have shaken hands, or contacted a creature after you've contacted a basic food item truck, etc.

Procedures to utilize hand sanitizer effectively:

Place the prescribed amount in the palm of one hand.

Rub your hands together, covering your whole hand.

Stop focusing on the sanitizer just once your skin is dry.

NOTE: Do not wipe off the hand sanitizer before it dries; it may not function properly against germs.

NOTE: Do NOT utilize hand sanitizer if your hands are filthy or oily: for instance, in the wake of cultivating, playing outside, or in the wake of outdoors (except if a handwashing station isn't accessible). Wash your hands with soap and water.

If you are making hand sanitizer at home, it is required to hold fast to these tips:

Make the hand sanitizer in a spotless space. Wipe down ledges with a weakened blanch arrangement beforehand.

Wash your hands completely before making the hand sanitizer.

To blend, utilize a spotless spoon and liquor. Wash these things completely before utilizing them.

Make sure the alcohol utilized for the hand sanitizer isn't weakened.

Mix all the constituents completely until they are very much mixed homogenously.

Do not contact the blend with your hands until it is prepared for use.

COMPELLING USES OF HAND SANITIZERS

Spot a modest quantity, (about the size of your thumbnail) on the palm of your hand. Rub it over your whole hand and your nail beds. You would realize that you have not utilized enough if the gel dissipates in under 15 seconds.

What To Look Out For?

The alcohol substance of hand chemicals might be as ethyl alcohol, ethanol, or isopropanol. Regardless of which kind of alcohol is recorded, its focus ought to be somewhere in the range of 60 and 95 percent. Anything short of 60 percent isn't sufficient to be a compelling chemical. While the utilization of alcohol is normal, a few gatherings have supported keeping alcohol-based ones from kids. They may lick the gels, and this can cause alcohol harming!

Maintain a strategic distance from 'without alcohol' sanitizers as there isn't a lot of information on those, and they can fluctuate in viability. It is made known that alcohol eliminates germs.

ADEQUACY OF ETHANOL AGAINST INFECTIONS IN HAND SANITIZATION

Ethanol is broadly utilized in hand rubs, gels, and froths for hand hygiene in healthcare settings. The World Health Organization has even recorded ethanol at 80% (v/v) as a basic medication in the classification 'alcohol-based hand rub. Since around the year 1994, the US Food and Drug Administration considers ethanol somewhere in the range of 60% and 95% as for the most part, sheltered and viable for hand scouring.

CLEANING AND SANITIZING YOUR BOTTLES/HOLDERS FOR YOUR HOMEMADE HAND SANITIZER.

The time has come to clean and purify the containers before packaging your custom made hand sanitizer. This is significant because your sanitizer gets awful if your container and equipment are grimy in any capacity - so ensure this is done appropriately.

First, ensure the container or compartment is perfect. Put the jug in a shower with water for about 20 to 30 minutes for the paste to break down. At that point, rub off the mark. In the event that it is hard to evacuate by hand, at that point, utilize the unpleasant side of a kitchen wipe to get it off.

While disinfecting, put around 40 ml of hydrogen peroxide 35% and then water in the sink. At that point, fill the spotless container in the sink, and let them be in the sink for 30 seconds. At that point, shake the containers with hydrogen peroxide of 35% and water in them, to ensure that all surfaces of the container are purified.

COULD A HAND SANITIZER (ALCOHOL TYPE) SUBSTITUTE FOR HANDWASHING?

Most of the alcohol-based sanitizers in the world contain ethanol or isopropanol or a mix of these two items. Most brands additionally contain a moisturizer to limit aggravation to the skin. Alcohol works promptly and adequately to eliminate microscopic organisms and most infections. The antimicrobial action of alcohol is its capacity to change proteins in microorganisms. Proteins and fats on ruined hands will diminish the viability of alcohol as a sanitizer. Alcohol arrangements containing 60%–95% of alcohol are the best. Higher focuses are less intense because proteins are not denatured effectively without water. Alcohol gels work by stripping the external layer of oil ceaselessly on the skin, in this manner, decimating any transient microorganisms present on the outside of the hands. After use, regrowth of microscopic organisms on the skin will, in general, happen gradually, in this manner, adequately keeping "remaining" microflora that dwells in more profound layers of skin from rising to the top. To be best, a dime-size touch of alcohol gel ought to be scoured into the hands for 30 seconds. On the off chance that hands are dry after just 10–15 seconds, all things considered, it is obvious that insufficient sanitizer was utilized.

14. ALCOHOL BASED SANITIZER RECIPES

FLORAL SANITIZER

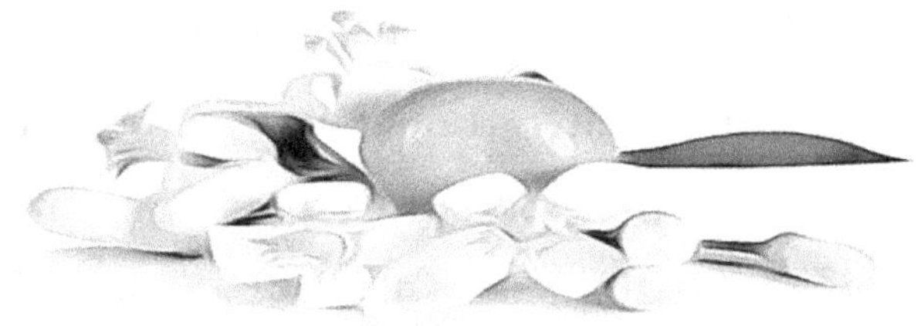

<u>Preparation Time</u>: 10 minutes

<u>Ingredients:</u>

- Isopropyl alcohol

- Witch hazel

- Orange blossom essential oil

<u>Directions:</u> This variation is going to be more like a spray, so make sure that you use the correct storage method. Whether you do not have any or you prefer to use something with a less sticky consistency, witch hazel is a very beneficial ingredient. It is normally used as a remedy for inflammation, infection, and skin damage. Not to mention, it has a naturally pleasant smell. Just as you did with the first recipe, mix 3

parts of alcohol with 1 part witch hazel (3:1). Add a few drops of orange blossom extract at the end for a lasting floral scent.

LAVENDER ESSENTIAL OIL HAND WASH

<u>Preparation time</u>: 20 minutes

<u>Ingredients:</u>

- ¾ cup of water
- ¼ cup of castile soap
- 20 drops of Lavender essential oil
- Soap dispenser

<u>Directions:</u>

Wash and rinse out any oil soap dispenser

Pour ¾ cups of water into the dispenser

Add ¼ cups of castile soap

Add 20 drops of lavender oil to the mixture

Place the dispenser lid and shake well

CINNAMON OIL SANITIZER

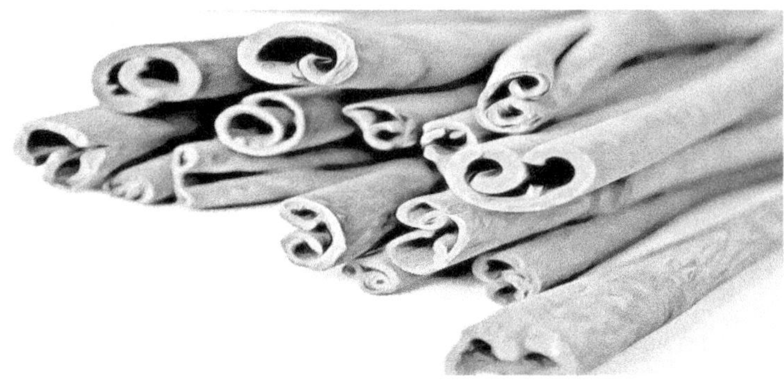

<u>Preparation time</u>: 10 minutes

<u>Ingredients</u>:

- 5 drops cinnamon essential oil

- 5 drops tea tree oil

- 1 tablespoon of rubbing alcohol

- ½ tablespoons aloe vera gel

- 2 cups boiled and cooled water

<u>Directions</u>:

In a glass bowl, add the essential oil, tree oil and rubbing alcohol and stir to combine.

Add the aloe vera gel and mix until well combined.

Now, add the water and mix until well combined.

Through a funnel, pour the hand sanitizer into small, clean squirt bottles.

Store in a cool place out of direct sunlight.

Remember to shake gently before each use.

THIEVES OIL HAND SANITIZER

<u>Preparation time</u>: 20 minutes

<u>Ingredients</u>:

- 9 tbsp (133 ml. / 4.5 fl. oz) isopropyl alcohol (99% rubbing alcohol)
- 3 tbsp (45 ml. / 1.5 fl. oz) 100% aloe vera gel
- 1 tbsp (15 ml. / 0.5 fl. oz) filtered water
- 10 drops vitamin E oil
- 10 drops vegetable glycerin
- 5 drops Thieves essential oil mixture

<u>Directions</u>:

Put the alcohol, aloe gel, water, vitamin E oil, and vegetable glycerin in a small bowl and mix well. Add the Thieves essential oil a few drops at a time, stirring slowly to combine. Store in a container of your choice. Shake before use.

HAND SANITIZER MADE WITH GALBANUM OIL AS THE ESSENTIAL OIL FOR FRAGRANCE

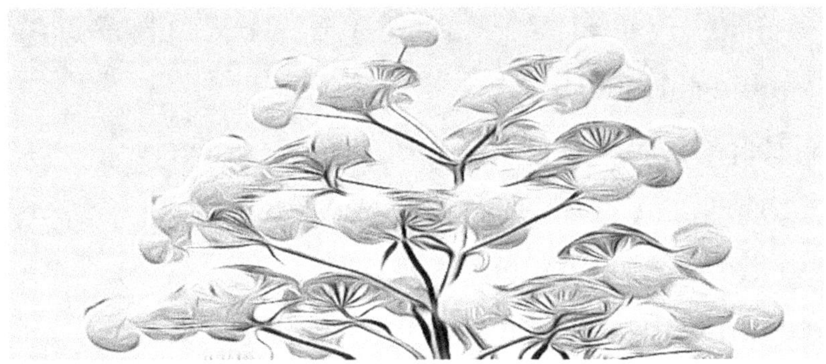

<u>Preparation Time</u>: 10 minutes

<u>Ingredients:</u>

- 15 drops of galbanum oil. (Galbanum essential oil has an earthy and woody scent that treats depression and stress. It also encourages circulation within the body.)
- 4 ounces of 99% rubbing alcohol.
- 2 ounces of aloe Vera gel.
- ¼ tablespoon of Vitamin E oil.

<u>Directions:</u>

Add 4 ounces of 99% rubbing alcohol to a clean bowl.

Add 2 ounces of aloe Vera gel to the bowl. Aloe Vera gel reduces the toxicity of alcohol to the hands. It also improves the quality of your skin.

Add 15 drops of the galbanum oil and ¼ tablespoon of the Vitamin E oil into the mix. The galbanum essential oil provides the scent for the hand sanitizer.

Using a clean spoon and a plastic paddle, stir the mixture until it is uniform. Clumping may occur due to aloe Vera gel. To eliminate it, you can stir vigorously for more than 60 seconds or blend the mixture.

Transfer the resulting combination into sterilized bottles and dispensers. You use a clean funnel to perform this action.

Label the sterilized bottles and dispensers so you can carry them wherever you go.

Clean your hands using the hand sanitizer.

HAND SANITIZER WITH SCHISANDRA OIL AS THE ESSENTIAL OIL

Preparation Time: 10 Minutes

Ingredients:

- 15 drops of schisandra essential oil. (Schisandra essential oil scent is known to uplift the mood of its users. It also improves concentration and can be used as an aphrodisiac.)
- 4 ounces of 99% isopropyl alcohol.
- 2 ounces of aloe Vera gel.
- ¼ tablespoon of vitamin E oil.

Directions:

Add 4 ounces of the 99% isopropyl alcohol to a clean bowl. You must also work in a clean space to prevent contamination of the ingredients or tools with germs such as bacteria and viruses.

Add 2 ounces of aloe Vera gel to the bowl. The aloe Vera gel provides the moisturizing effect of the hand sanitizer on the hands.

Put 15 drops of the schisandra essential oil and ¼ tablespoon of vitamin E oil to the bowl. The schisandra essential oil is responsible for the scent of the hand sanitizer. The vitamin E oil is responsible for reducing the toxicity of alcohol on the hands by covering the cracks on the hands.

Stir the ingredients thoroughly for over 60 seconds to avoid clumping. You can use a sterilized spoon or a whisk to perform this step.

Transfer the contents of the bowl into sterilized bottles and dispensers. Label the sterilized bottles and dispensers as hand sanitizers for easy identification.

Clean your hands using the hand sanitizers.

HAND SANITIZER USING YARROW OIL AS THE ESSENTIAL OIL FOR FRAGRANCE

Preparation Time: 10 minutes

Ingredients:

- 15 drops of yarrow essential oil. (Yarrow oil is used in perfumery because of its sweet smell. The scent has many benefits including relieving respiratory conditions, clearing your mind and reducing your depression.)

- 4 ounces of 99% isopropyl alcohol.
- 2 ounces of aloe Vera gel.
- ¼ tablespoon of Vitamin E essential oil

<u>Directions:</u>

Add 4 ounces of 99% isopropyl alcohol to a clean bowl.

Add 2 ounces of the aloe Vera gel to the bowl.

Put 15 drops of the yarrow essential oil and the ¼ tablespoon of vitamin E oil to the bowl. The yarrow essential oil creates the scent of the hand sanitizer. The vitamin E oil reduces the harshness of the alcohol towards the hand and the skin.

Beat the mixture using a sterilized whisk until the ingredients are uniformly combined. This action can take 60 to 70 seconds. You can sing a song while beating the ingredients to keep you concentrated.

Transfer the contents of the bowl into sterilized bottles and dispensers. If the bowl had a pouring spout, then you could easily fill the bottles and dispensers. However, clean funnels can also complete the action.

Label the bottles and dispensers as hand sanitizers.

Use the hand sanitizer to keep your hands clean.

HAND SANITIZER WITH RAVENSARA OIL AS THE ESSENTIAL OIL

<u>Preparation Time</u>: 10 minutes

<u>Ingredients:</u>

- 15 drops of ravensara essential oil. (Ravensara oil scent is used to treat respiratory conditions such as phlegm and increased mucus in the windpipe.)
- 4 ounces of 99% Isopropyl alcohol.
- 2 ounces of aloe Vera gel.
- ¼ tablespoon of vitamin E oil.

<u>Directions:</u>

Add 4 ounces of 99% alcohol into a sanitized bowl.

Add 2 ounces of the aloe Vera gel into the sanitized bowl.

Put 15 drops of the ravensara essential oil and ¼ tablespoon of the vitamin E oil. The ravensara essential oil will give the hand sanitizer its scent. The vitamin E oil will act as a moisturizer and work together with aloe Vera gel to reduce the toxicity of alcohol on your hands.

Mix the materials in the bowl using a clean plastic paddle or spoon for about 40 to 60 seconds.

Pour the mixture into sterilized bottles and dispensers. Label these containers as hand sanitizers for easy identification.

Clean your hands using this hand sanitizer.

HYDROGEN PEROXIDE SANITIZER

<u>Preparation time</u>: 10 minutes

<u>Ingredients:</u> 1 cup rubbing alcohol

- 1 tablespoon 3% hydrogen peroxide
- 1 teaspoon aloe vera gel
- Boiled and cooled water, as required

<u>Directions:</u>

In a glass bowl, add the rubbing alcohol and hydrogen peroxide and stir to combine.

Add the aloe vera gel and mix until well combined.

Now, add the enough water that brings the total liquid to 11/3 cups and mix until well combined.

Through a funnel, pour the hand sanitizer into small, clean squirt bottles.

Store in a cool place out of direct sunlight.

Remember to shake gently before each use.

HYDROGEN PEROXIDE & GLYCERIN SANITIZER

<u>Preparation time</u>: 10 minutes

<u>Ingredients:</u>

- 5 drops tea tree essential oil
- 1 2/3 cups rubbing alcohol
- 1 tablespoon 3% hydrogen peroxide
- 2 teaspoons glycerin
- ¼ cup distilled water

Directions:

In a glass bowl, add the essential oil, rubbing alcohol and hydrogen peroxide and stir to combine.

Add the glycerin and mix until well combined.

Now, add the water and mix until well combined.

Through a funnel, pour the hand sanitizer into small, clean squirt bottles.

Store in a cool place out of direct sunlight.

Remember to shake gently before each use.

EUCALYPTUS OIL SANITIZER

Preparation time: 10 minutes

Ingredients:

- 2/3 cup rubbing alcohol
- 10 drops eucalyptus essential oil
- 1/3 cup aloe vera gel

Directions:

In a glass bowl, add the rubbing alcohol and essential oil and stir to combine.

Add the aloe vera gel and mix until well combined.

Through a funnel, pour the hand sanitizer into small, clean squirt bottles.

Store in a cool place out of direct sunlight.

Remember to shake gently before each use.

EUCALYPTUS & TEA TREE OIL SANITIZER

<u>Preparation time</u>: 10 minutes

<u>Ingredients</u>:

- 15 drops eucalyptus essential oil
- 5 drops tea tree oil
- 1 tablespoon rubbing alcohol
- ½ tablespoons aloe vera gel
- 2 cups boiled and cooled water

<u>Directions</u>:

In a glass bowl, add the essential oil, tree oil and rubbing alcohol and stir to combine.

Add the aloe vera gel and mix until well combined.

Now, add the water and mix until well combined.

Through a funnel, pour the hand sanitizer into small, clean squirt bottles.

Store in a cool place out of direct sunlight.

Remember to shake gently before each use.

15. NON ALCOHOL HAND SANITIZER RECIPES

ALOE VERA-FREE SANITIZER

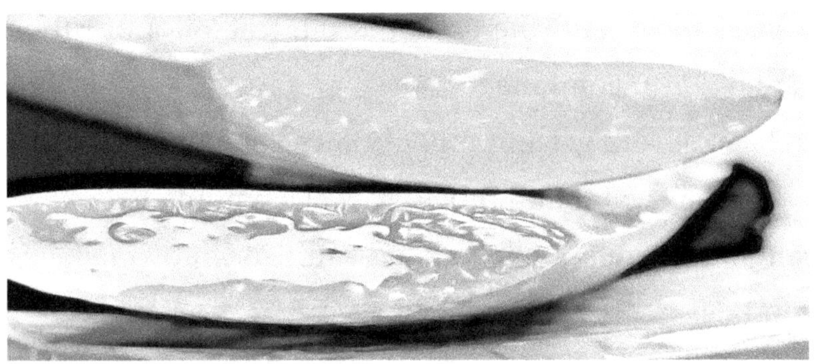

<u>Preparation time</u>: 10 minutes

Ingredients:

- 2 tablespoons vodka
- 5 drops orange essential oil
- 5 drops lemon essential oil
- 2 drops Vitamin E oil
- 5 drops tea tree oil
- Sterile water, as required

Directions:

In a glass bowl, add the essential oils and rubbing alcohol and stir to combine.

Fill a small, clean squirt bottle most of the way with sterile water.

Through a funnel, pour the hand sanitizer into small, clean squirt bottles.

Store in a cool place out of direct sunlight.

Remember to shake gently before each use.

PURE ALOE VERA & ROSEMARY OIL SANITIZER

Preparation time: 10 minutes

Ingredients:

- ½ cup aloe vera juice
- ¼ cup vodka
- 10-20 drops rosemary essential oil
- 1 tablespoon organic lavender lotion

Directions:

In a glass bowl, add the aloe vera juice, vodka, essential oil and lavender lotion and mix until well combined.

Through a funnel, pour the hand sanitizer into small, clean squirt bottles.

Store in a cool place out of direct sunlight.

Remember to shake gently before each use.

VITAMIN E & LAVENDER OIL SANITIZER

<u>Preparation time</u>: 10 minutes

<u>Ingredients</u>:

- 30 drops tea tree essential oil
- 5-10 drops lavender essential oil
- ¼ teaspoon Vitamin E oil
- 3 ounces high-proof vodka
- 1 ounce pure aloe vera gel

<u>Directions</u>:

In a glass bowl, add both essential oils, Vitamin E oil and vodka and stir to combine.

Add the aloe vera gel and mix until well combined.

Through a funnel, pour the hand sanitizer into small, clean squirt bottles.

Store in a cool place out of direct sunlight.

Remember to shake gently before each use.

LEMONGRASS OIL SANITIZER

<u>Preparation time</u>: 10 minutes

<u>Ingredients</u>:

- ½ cup aloe vera juice
- ¼ cup vodka
- 15-20 drops lemongrass essential oil
- 1 tablespoon vegetable glycerin

<u>Directions</u>:

In a glass bowl, add the aloe vera juice, vodka and essential oil and mix until well combined.

Add the vegetable glycerin and mix until well combined.

Through a funnel, pour the hand sanitizer into small, clean squirt bottles.

Store in a cool place out of direct sunlight.

Remember to shake gently before each use.

THYME OIL SANITIZER

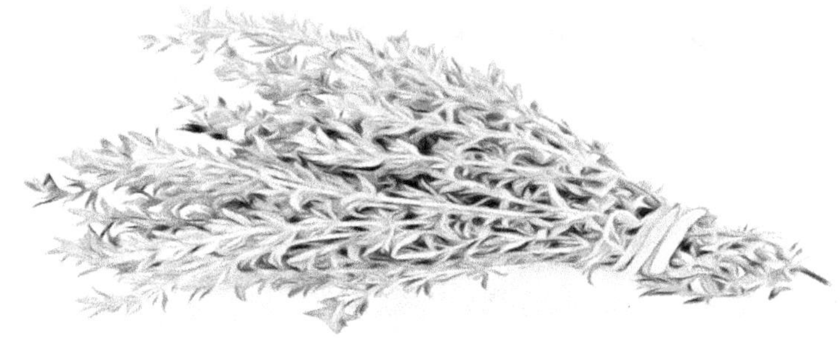

<u>Preparation time</u>: 10 minutes

<u>Ingredients</u>:

- ½ cup aloe vera juice
- ¼ cup vodka
- 15-20 drops thyme essential oil
- 1 tablespoon organic lavender lotion
- 1 tablespoon vegetable glycerin

<u>Directions</u>:

In a glass bowl, add the aloe vera juice, vodka, essential oil and lavender lotion and mix until well combined.

Add the vegetable glycerin and mix until well combined.

Through a funnel, pour the hand sanitizer into small, clean squirt bottles.

Store in a cool place out of direct sunlight.

Remember to shake gently before each use.

3 OILS SANITIZER

<u>Preparation time</u>: 10 minutes

<u>Ingredients</u>:

- 30 drops tea tree essential oil
- 5-10 drops lavender essential oil
- ¼ teaspoon Vitamin E oil
- 3 ounces high-proof vodka
- 1 ounce pure aloe vera gel

<u>Directions</u>:

In a glass bowl, add both essential oils, Vitamin E oil and vodka and stir to combine.

Add the aloe vera gel and mix until well combined.

Through a funnel, pour the hand sanitizer into small, clean squirt bottles.

Store in a cool place out of direct sunlight.

Remember to shake gently before each use.

4 OILS SANITIZER

<u>Preparation time</u>: 10 minutes

<u>Ingredients</u>:

- 10 drops lavender essential oil
- 5 drops lemongrass essential oil
- 20 drops tea tree oil
- 1 teaspoon Vitamin E oil solution

- 4 tablespoons vodka
- 2 tablespoons aloe vera gel

Directions:

In a glass bowl, add both essential oils, tree oil, Vitamin E oil solution and vodka and stir to combine.

Add the aloe vera gel and mix until well combined.

Through a funnel, pour the hand sanitizer into small, clean squirt bottles.

Store in a cool place out of direct sunlight.

Remember to shake gently before each use.

GLYCERIN & 4 OILS SANITIZER

Preparation time: 10 minutes

Ingredients:

- 2 drops eucalyptus essential oil
- 2 drops rosemary essential oil
- 2 drops cinnamon leaf essential oil
- 2 drops clove bud essential oil
- 2 tablespoons vodka
- 1 teaspoon aloe vera juice
- ½ teaspoon vegetable glycerin
- 2 tablespoons sterile water

Directions:

In a glass bowl, add all oils, vodka and aloe vera juice and stir to combine.

Add the vegetable glycerin and mix until well combined.

Now, add the water and mix until well combined.

Through a funnel, pour the hand sanitizer into small, clean squirt bottles.

Store in a cool place out of direct sunlight.

Remember to shake gently before each use.

EUCALYPTUS OIL SANITIZER

<u>Preparation time</u>: 10 minutes

<u>Ingredients</u>:

- ¼ cup vodka
- 15 drops eucalyptus essential oil
- 1 tablespoon organic lavender lotion
- ½ cup aloe vera gel
- 1 tablespoon vegetable glycerin

<u>Directions</u>:

In a glass bowl, add the vodka, essential oil and lavender lotion and mix until well combined.

Add the aloe vera gel and vegetable glycerin and mix until well combined.

Through a funnel, pour the hand sanitizer into small, clean squirt bottles.

Store in a cool place out of direct sunlight.

Remember to shake gently before each use.

LAVENDER & LEMONGRASS OIL SANITIZER

Preparation time: 10 minutes

Ingredients:

- 1 teaspoon Vitamin E oil
- 10 drops lavender essential oil
- 6 drops lemongrass essential oil
- 25 drops tea tree oil
- 12 teaspoons witch hazel
- 6 teaspoons aloe vera gel

Directions:

In a glass bowl, add all the Vitamin E oil, essential oils and tree oil and witch hazel and stir to combine.

Add the aloe vera gel and mix until well combined.

Through a funnel, pour the hand sanitizer into small, clean squirt bottles.

Store in a cool place out of direct sunlight.

Remember to shake gently before each use.

CLOVE OIL SANITIZER

Preparation time: 10 minutes

Ingredients:

- ¼ cup witch hazel
- 10-20 drops clove essential oil

- 1 tablespoon organic lavender lotion
- ½ cup aloe vera gel
- 1 tablespoon vegetable glycerin

Instructions:

In a glass bowl, add the witch hazel, essential oil and lavender lotion and mix until well combined.

Add the aloe vera gel and vegetable glycerin and mix until well combined.

Through a funnel, pour the hand sanitizer into small, clean squirt bottles.

Store in a cool place out of direct sunlight.

Remember to shake gently before each use.

CINNAMON OIL SANITIZER

Preparation time: 10 minutes

Ingredients: ¼ cup witch hazel

- 15-20 drops cinnamon essential oil ½ cup aloe vera gel

Directions:

In a glass bowl, add the witch hazel and essential oil and mix until well combined.

Add the aloe vera gel and mix until well combined.

Through a funnel, pour the hand sanitizer into small, clean squirt bottles.

Store in a cool place out of direct sunlight.

Remember to shake gently before each use.

CASTILE SOAP & TEA TREE OIL SANITIZER

<u>Preparation time</u>: 10 minutes

<u>Ingredients</u>: 10 drops tea tree essential oil

- 1 teaspoon castile soap
- 6 ounces boiled and cooled water

<u>Instructions</u>: In a glass bowl, add the essential oil and castile soap and stir to combine. Now, add the water and mix until well combined. Through a funnel, pour the hand sanitizer into small, clean squirt bottles.

Store in a cool place out of direct sunlight.

Remember to shake gently before each use.

16.   DIY HAND SANITIZER GEL RECIPES (How To Make)

QUICK SANITIZING GEL

<u>Preparation time</u>: 20 minutes

<u>Ingredients</u>: Isopropyl alcohol

- Aloe vera gel
- Tea tree oil
- 15 ml carrageenan
- 50 ml of distilled water
- 10 g of vegetable glycerin
- 50 ml food grade alcohol
- 7 drops of scotch pine essential oil

<u>Directions:</u>

Pour the water into a glass and add the carrageenan.

Stir well and let the solution rest until it has formed a gel.

In another glass pour the food grade alcohol, add the glycerin and the essential oils. Mix gently Add the alcohol solution to the gel and stir slowly.

When you need something quick, this recipe will allow you to create a hand sanitizer gel that requires very few ingredients. Start by mixing 3 parts isopropyl alcohol with 1 part aloe vera gel. Depending on how much you need to make, you can use your best judgment on the proportions. Add a few drops of tea tree oil for a pleasant lasting scent and anti-inflammatory properties.

SCOTCH PINE ESSENTIAL OIL GEL

Transfer to a clean dry bottle and store the product away from direct sources of light and keep for a maximum of three months.

CHAMOMILE OIL GEL RECIPE

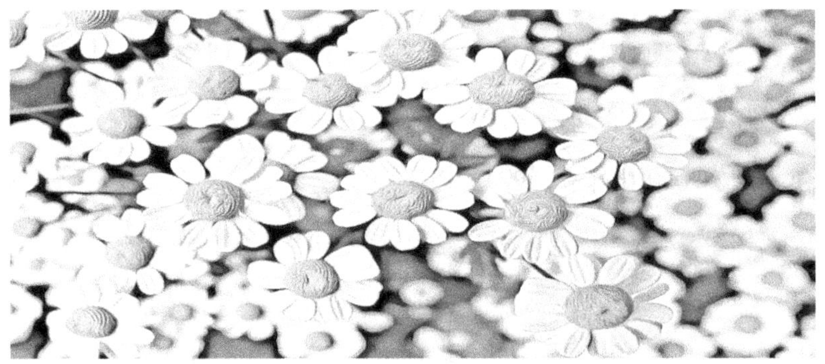

<u>Preparation Time:</u> 20 minutes

<u>Ingredients:</u>

- 2 cups of water

- 5 drops of Tea tree oil
- 15 drops of Chamomile essential oil
- ½ tablespoons of Aloe Vera gel
- 1 tablespoon of Rubbing alcohol

Directions:

To produce Chamomile fragranced hand sanitizer, pour and mix all listed ingredients together in a bowl and stir well. Blend the mixture well and pure then into any container for future use.

LEMON OIL GEL RECIPE

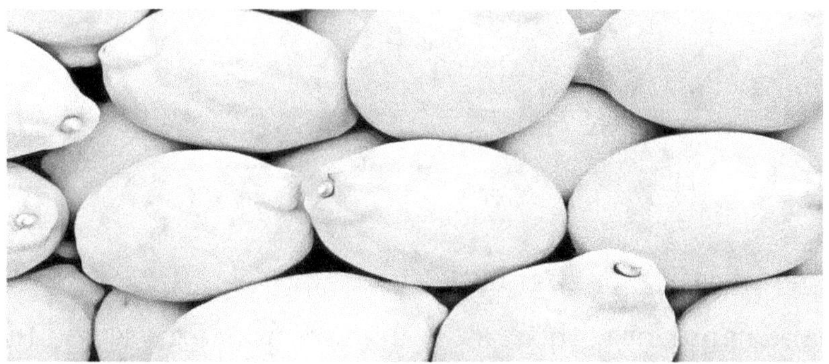

Preparation Time: 20 minutes

Lemon has a widely accepted and favored fragrance, which give a refreshing feeling to the users. To produce your homemade lemon fragrance, follow below detailed steps.

Ingredients:

- 2 cups of water
- 5 drops of Tea tree oil

- 5 drops of lemon essential oil
- ½ tablespoons of Aloe Vera gel
- 1 tablespoon of Rubbing alcohol

<u>Directions:</u>

To produce Lemon fragranced hand sanitizer, pour and mix all listed ingredients together in a bowl and stir well. Blend the mixture well and pure then into any container for future use.

SWEET ORANGE FLAVOR GEL RECIPE

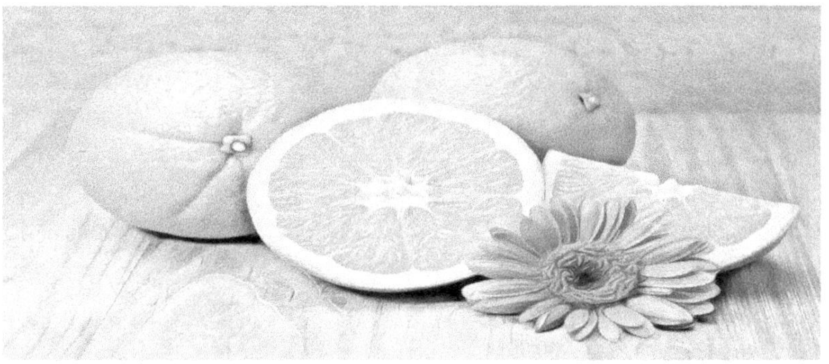

<u>Preparation Time:</u> 20 minutes

A hand sanitizer with sweet orange fragrance gives you that needed energetic feeling with the smell and keeps you happy.

<u>Ingredients:</u>

- 2 cups of water
- 5 drops of Tea tree oil
- 15 drops of Sweet Orange essential oil
- ½ tablespoons of Aloe Vera gel
- 1 tablespoon of Rubbing alcohol

<u>Directions</u>:

To produce Sweet Orange fragranced hand sanitizer, pour and mix all listed ingredients together in a bowl and stir well. Blend the mixture well and pure then into any container for future use.

ALOE VERA GEL

<u>Preparation Time</u>: 10 minutes

This forms a base gel, and aloe is very nourishing to the skin.

Isopropyl Alcohol 91%-Make sure that the final product is 91% (not 70%) to achieve the required concentration in WHO and CDC.

Essential oils-Tea tree oil has strong antibacterial properties (using a concentration of at least 0.5%), and lavender rounds off the strong smell of tea tree oil. You can also use thyme oil, which has been shown to be effective against drug-resistant bacteria.

Vitamin E Oil-acts as a natural moisturizer for the skin and counteracts the hardness of alcohol.

This is the type of alcohol you need. Make sure the hand sanitizer is at least 91% to reach the minimum alcohol level required by the World Health Organization.

<u>Ingredients</u>:

- 1 cup 91% isopropyl alcohol (do not use 70% as this will change the concentration)
- 1/2 cup aloe vera gel
- 45 drops of tea tree oil (optional, additional antibacterial)
- 15 drops of essential oil (rosemary, lavender and cinnamon are the best way to end it)
- 3/4 tsp vitamin E oil (optional, for moisturizing)
- Squeeze tube or bottle

<u>Directions</u>:

Put the essential oil and vitamin E oil in a small glass bowl and stir.

Add alcohol and stir again.

Add aloe vera gel and mix well.

Adopting a pipe, splash the disorder within the picked container.

Shake well before use

ALMOND OIL SANITIZER

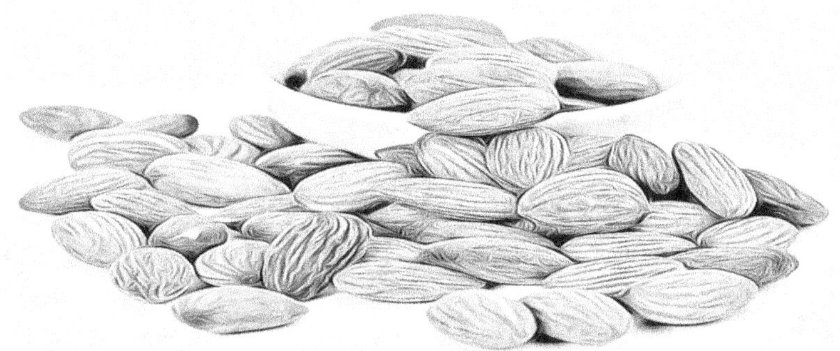

Preparation time: 10 minutes

Ingredients: 30 drops tea tree essential oil

- 10 drops lavender essential oil ¼ teaspoon almond oil
- 1 tablespoon witch hazel extract 1 cup aloe vera gel

Directions:

In a glass bowl, add the essential oils, almond oil and witch hazel extract and stir to combine.

Add the aloe vera gel and mix until well combined.

Through a funnel, pour the hand sanitizer into small, clean squirt bottles. Store in a cool place out of direct sunlight.

Remember to shake gently before each use.

GERM DESTROYER & VITAMIN E OIL SANITIZER

Preparation time: 10 minutes

Ingredients:

- ¼ teaspoon vitamin E oil

- 35 drops Germ Destroyer essential oil
- 1 tablespoon witch hazel solution
- 1 tablespoon aloe vera gel

<u>Directions</u>:

In a glass bowl, add the vitamin E oil, Germ Destroyer and witch hazel solution and stir to combine.

Add the aloe vera gel and mix until well combined.

Through a funnel, pour the hand sanitizer into small, clean squirt bottles.

Store in a cool place out of direct sunlight.

Remember to shake gently before each use.

PEPPERMINT OIL SANITIZER

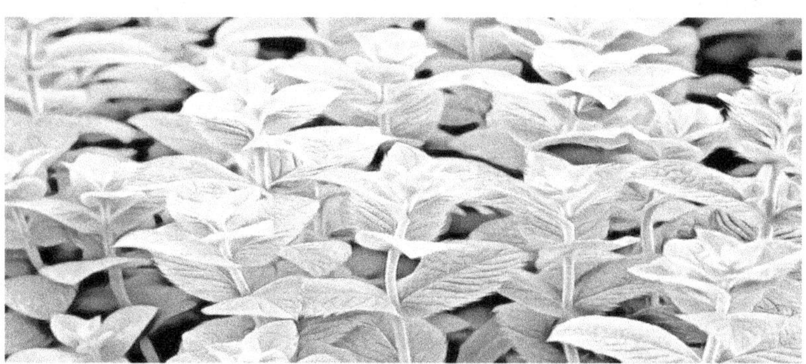

<u>Preparation time</u>: 10 minutes

<u>Ingredients</u>:

- 5 drops peppermint essential oil
- 30 drops tea tree oil
- 1½ teaspoons witch hazel

- 1 cup pure aloe vera gel

<u>Directions</u>:

In a glass bowl, add the essential oil, tree oil and witch hazel and witch hazel and stir to combine.

Add the aloe vera gel and mix until well combined.

Through a funnel, pour the hand sanitizer into small, clean squirt bottles.

Store in a cool place out of direct sunlight.

Remember to shake gently before each use.

ROSEMARY OIL SANITIZER

<u>Preparation time</u>: 10 minutes

<u>Ingredients</u>:

- 30 drops tea tree oil
- 5-10 drops rosemary essential oil
- 2 tablespoon witch hazel
- 1 cup aloe vera gel

<u>Directions</u>:

In a glass bowl, add the tree oil, essential oil and witch hazel and mix until well combined.

Add the aloe vera gel and mix until well combined.

Through a funnel, pour the hand sanitizer into small, clean squirt bottles.

Store in a cool place out of direct sunlight.

Remember to shake gently before each use.

17.   DIY HAND SANITIZER SPRAY RECIPES

MOISTURIZING SANITIZER (GEL OR SPRAY)

<u>Preparation Time</u>: 10 minutes

<u>Ingredients</u>: Lavender oil - Tea tree oil

- Isopropyl alcohol
- Aloe vera gel OR witch hazel
- Vitamin E oil

<u>Directions</u>:

This recipe gives you many options and benefits. To begin, decide whether you want to make a gel or a spray: this will indicate whether you should use aloe vera gel or witch hazel. After obtaining the proper storage methods, you can begin by combining 5-10 drops of lavender oil, 30 drops of tea tree oil, 3 ounces of isopropyl alcohol, 1 ounce of aloe vera gel or witch hazel, and ¼ teaspoon of vitamin E oil in a bowl. This recipe allows you to make a bigger batch, suitable for most families. You will be able to fill 5 spray bottles or 5 containers when you use these proportions. It is important to consider recipes like this one that can allow you to make enough for your entire family in one sitting. This recipe provides a very convenient and effective way to keep your hands clean while also receiving the benefits of the added scents and moisturizing vitamin E oil. This sanitizer will help make your hands look and smell great, while simultaneously keeping them clean.

CITRUS SANITIZER SPRAY

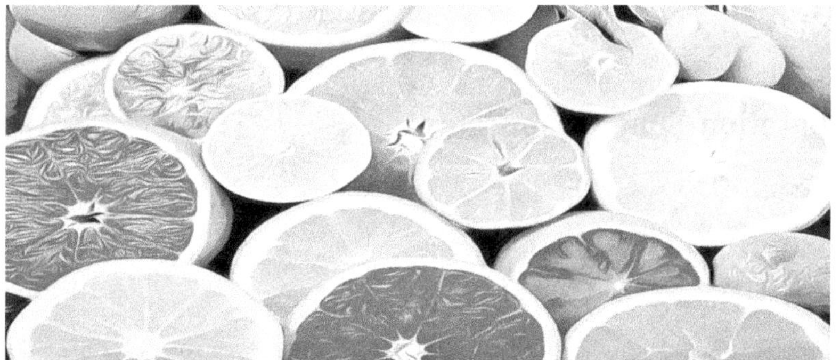

<u>Preparation Time</u>: 10 minutes

<u>Ingredients</u>: Vitamin E oil

- Lemon essential oil

- Orange essential oil

- Tea tree oil

- Witch hazel with aloe vera

- Isopropyl alcohol

- Distilled water

<u>Directions</u>:

Combine 5 drops of vitamin E oil, 3 tablespoons of witch hazel, 5 drops of lemon oil, 5 drops of orange oil, 5 drops of tea tree oil, 5 tablespoons of isopropyl alcohol in your spray bottle. Shake the bottle to mix all of the ingredients together.

Once mixed, fill the rest of the bottle to the top with distilled water. This is a fragrant recipe that will leave behind a refreshing citrus scent that you can enjoy. It will also keep your hands soft without you having to rely on using a moisturizer after each time you sanitize your hands with the spray.

SANITIZING SPRAY

<u>Preparation Time</u>: 10 minutes

<u>Ingredients</u>:

- Isopropyl alcohol
- Glycerin or glycerol
- Hydrogen peroxide
- Distilled water
- Spray bottle

<u>Directions</u>:

Some people prefer their hand sanitizer to come in a spray form because it is less messy. It also encourages you to use less product as you must spritz your hands rather than apply gel on them. This recipe does not contain aloe, which some people find to be sticky after use. To start, mix 12 fluid oz of alcohol with 2 teaspoons of glycerin/glycerol. The latter helps to prevent the alcohol from drying out your hands, so it is an essential ingredient in this recipe. If you cannot find any, you can still proceed with the recipe and remember to moisturize your hands well after using the spray. Continue by mixing in 1 teaspoon of hydrogen peroxide and 3 fluid oz of distilled water. If you do not have distilled water, you can improvise by boiling water and then allowing it to cool completely before use.

FIR NEEDLE SANITIZER RECIPE

Preparation Time: 10 minutes

Fir needle essential oil cleansing and healing oil in your regular blends and aromatherapy preparations long after the seasonal fires have cooled.

Ingredients: 2 cups of water 5 drops of Tea tree oil

- 15 drops of Fir needle essential oil
- ½ tablespoons of Aloe Vera gel
- 1 tablespoon of Rubbing alcohol

Directions:

To produce Fir Needle fragranced hand sanitizer, pour and mix all listed ingredients together in a bowl and stir well. Blend the mixture well and pure then into any container for future use.

BALSAM FIR SANITIZER RECIPE

<u>Preparation Time</u>: 10 minutes

Balsam Fir Essential Oil helps support a healthy respiratory system. Additionally, Balsam Fir is widely used by many for its emotional balancing and soothing effects on the skin

<u>Ingredients:</u>

- 2 cups of water
- 5 drops of Tea tree oil
- 15 drops of Balsam Fir essential oil
- ½ tablespoons of Aloe Vera gel
- 1 tablespoon of Rubbing alcohol

<u>Directions:</u>

To produce Balsam Fir fragranced hand sanitizer, pour and mix all listed ingredients together in a bowl and stir well. Blend the mixture well and pure then into any container for future use.

DOUGLAS FIR SANITIZER RECIPE

<u>Preparation Time</u>: 10 minutes

<u>Ingredients:</u>

- 2 cups of water
- 5 drops of Tea tree oil
- 15 drops of Douglas Fir essential oil
- ½ tablespoons of Aloe Vera gel

- 1 tablespoon of Rubbing alcohol

<u>Directions:</u>

To produce Douglas Fir fragranced hand sanitizer, pour and mix all listed ingredients together in a bowl and stir well. Blend the mixture well and pure then into any container for future use. To produce Douglas Fir fragranced hand sanitizer, pour and mix all listed ingredients together in a bowl and stir well. Blend the mixture well and pure then into any container for future use.

WHITE FIR SANITIZER RECIPE

<u>Preparation Time:</u> 10 minutes

<u>Ingredients:</u>

- 2 cups of water
- 5 drops of Tea tree oil
- 15 drops of White Fir essential oil
- ½ tablespoons of Aloe Vera gel
- 1 tablespoon of Rubbing alcohol

<u>Directions:</u>

To produce White Fir fragranced hand sanitizer, pour and mix all listed ingredients together in a bowl and stir well. Blend the mixture well and pure then into any container for future use.

PEPPERMINT SANITIZER RECIPE

<u>Preparation Time</u>: 10 minutes

Peppermint is known as a combination or hybrid of spearmint and water mint that is naturally grown. The flower and leaves are harvested to extract the essential oil from them.

<u>Ingredients:</u>

- 2 cups of water
- 5 drops of Tea tree oil
- 15 drops of Peppermint essential oil
- ½ tablespoons of Aloe Vera gel
- 1 tablespoon of Rubbing alcohol

<u>Directions:</u>

To produce Peppermint fragranced hand sanitizer, pour and mix all listed ingredients together in a bowl and stir well. Blend the mixture well and pure then into any container for future use.

VANILLA SANITIZER RECIPE

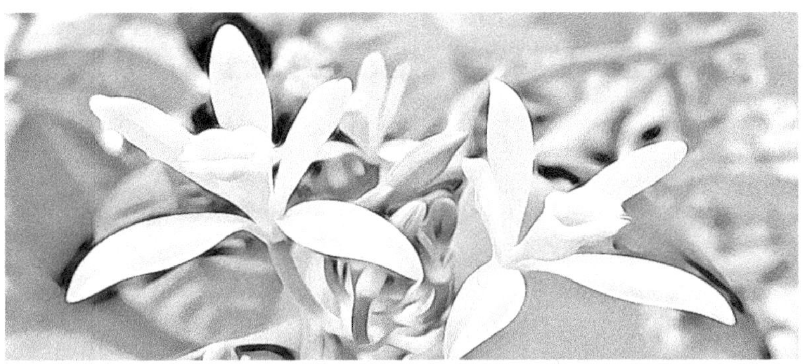

<u>Preparation Time</u>: 10 minutes

Use Vanilla Essential oil for a pleasant-smelling and yet effective in its anti-bacterial functions. You can combine it with citrus to an added boost and a refreshing blend of scent

<u>Ingredients</u>:

- 2 cups of water
- 5 drops of Tea tree oil
- 15 drops of Vanilla essential oil
- ½ tablespoons of Aloe Vera gel
- 1 tablespoon of Rubbing alcohol

<u>Directions</u>:

To produce Vanilla hand sanitizer, pour and mix all listed ingredients together in a bowl and stir well. Blend the mixture well and pure then into any container for future use.

18.   DIY DISINFECTANT SURFACE WIPES

HOMEMADE DISINFECTANT WIPES

Basic Disinfectant Wipes:

Equipment

1.) Glass Jar

2.) 10 Washcloths

3.) Pot or Pan

4.) Scissors

5.) Bowl

<u>Ingredients:</u>

1.) 3 cups Boiled water (cooled down)

2.) ¾ Cup Rubbing Alcohol

3.) 6 tsp Dawn Dish soap

4.) 10 Drops Lemon Essential Oil

<u>Directions:</u> Before starting like many of the other recipes here put some water into a pot or pan of your choice. Set the chosen pot or pan on the stove to boil for 5 to 10 minutes. Afterwards set the pan aside to cool. This will be the boiled

water used later in the recipe. Now you can begin prepping the cleaning solution and wipes.

First cut your washcloths to the desired size using scissors. Generally, the washcloths are cut in half. Once the cloths are cut to the desired size, fill the jar with the washcloths.

In a bowl, Mix the boiled water, rubbing alcohol, dish soap, and essential oil together. Stir this solution until it is uniform. Pour this into the jar that contains all the washcloths and let them soak. Close up the jar when you are finished. The washcloths are ready to be used for any cleaning purpose as they are needed.

Notes and Safety

Rubbing Alcohol

When handling rubbing alcohol, it is important not to swallow any or get any in your eyes. Rubbing alcohol is toxic when ingested. Make sure to only use it in an area that has good ventilation and that you NEVER mix rubbing alcohol with bleach. Mixing rubbing alcohol with bleach creates chloroform which is a toxic substance so it should always be avoided.

Notes

Once the cleaning rags get dirty, they can be washed in a washing machine as you normally would. After this they can be remade into the same sanitizing wipes, they once were by repeating the recipe a second time

The jar that contains the rags is best if it is made of glass. Essential oils tend to react with plastic containers and a side reaction is not desired when creating disinfectant wipes.

VINEGAR BASED DISINFECTANT WIPES:

Equipment:

1.) Pot or pan

2.) Mason Jar or other container

3.) Washcloths

4.) Scissors

5.) Bowl

Ingredients:

1.) ¾ Cup Boiled water (Cooled Down)

2.) ¾ Cup Distilled Vinegar

3.) 15 Drops Lemon Essential Oil

4.) 8 Drops Lavender Essential Oil

5.) 4 Drops Bergamot Essential Oil

Directions:

Add water to the pot or pan. Bring it to a boil on a stovetop for 5 to 10 minutes. After this set the water aside to cool. This will be the water that is used in the solution later in the recipe.

Cut the washcloths up into the size desired. Generally, these are cut in half. Place them into the mason jar or other container. Add the water, essential oils, and vinegar to a bowl. Mix these until the solution becomes uniform. Add the solution to the jar that contains the wipes. Close the lid of the jar and let the wipes soak. Store until they need to be used.

Notes and Safety

Essential Oils

Undiluted essential oils can burn and be poisonous if swallowed. Be sure not to ingest any or get any on your skin while preparing the sanitizer. Once the oils are diluted in the mixture, they should be safe.

Notes:

Once the cleaning rags get dirty, they can be washed in a washing machine as you normally would. After this they can be remade into the same sanitizing wipes, they once were by repeating the recipe a second time.

HOMEMADE ALCOHOL AND SOAP BASED CLEANING WIPES RECIPE

<u>Preparation Time</u>: 10 minutes

<u>Ingredients</u>:

- 2 cups of distilled water
- ¼ cup of rubbing alcohol
- 1 teaspoon of dish soap
- 20 drops of essential oil blend

<u>TOOLS</u>:

- Quart – sized mason jar
- 16 small thin clothes (size approximately 8-10 inches)

<u>Directions</u>:

Take your jar and add ¼ cup of rubbing alcohol, 2 cups distilled water and 20 drops of essential oil blend. Put the lid on shake gently in order to mix properly.

When you are done mixing, remove the lid from the jar and put your cleaning clothes into it. Proceed by adding them till the cleaning solution has absorbed into the clothes. Put again the lid on the jar and then turn it upside down for a couple of minutes. Now your wipes are ready to be used.

Once you've used all your wipes, collect them in a container and when you want to make another batch, just wash them with your laundry and use them again.

HOMEMADE WATER, VINEGAR AND ALCOHOL BASED CLEANING WIPES RECIPE

The following recipe also suggests a safer and natural way to make your chemical-free homemade wipes by using vinegar, water and alcohol.

Let's have a look.

<u>Preparation Time</u>: 10 minutes

<u>Ingredients</u>:

- 1 cup distilled water
- 1/2 cup vinegar (white distilled vinegar if possible)
- 1/4 cup rubbing alcohol
- 12 drops lavender essential oil
- 8 drops orange or lemon essential oil
- 8 drops tea tree oil
- 5 drops peppermint essential oil

<u>Tools</u>:

- 20 small thin clothes (size approximately 8-10 inches)
- Quart – sized mason jar

<u>Directions</u>:

Take your container and add to it 1 cup of distilled water, ½ cup of vinegar and ¼ cup of rubbing alcohol. Stir these ingredients altogether. Now add all the essential oils and stir altogether in order to combine them. Then add the thin clothes to the container and put it upside down, in this way all the clothes will absorb properly all the solution. Leave it for a couple of minutes. Your wipes are finally ready to be used.

Conclusions

Hand sanitizer is an effective and readily available means of stemming the explosion of bacterial and viral infection and is particularly effective for personal protection. Hand sanitizers do go a long way in helping to safeguard you.

In the event that your local supermarket or store is out of hand sanitizer, you can conveniently use this guide to produce one for personal and household use. The required ingredients aren't much and could be readily gotten. All you basically need to create one of these highly-essential virus combatants is isopropyl alcohol, a cupful of aloe vera gel, and any essential of your choosing.

Regardless of the fact that hand sanitizers are useful tools for preventing germinal infections, health experts still endorse washing your hand washing every time it's feasible to better safeguard yourself from pathogens, viruses and other harmful microorganisms.

A typical error made when making use of a hand sanitizer is not sufficient. The hand sanitizer must be used with no less than a cent on the palms on the hands and rubbed. Cover all surfaces, which includes the palms, back of the hand, between the toes, around the nails as well as wrists, just like you will wash your hands. This is the only way that hand sanitizers thoroughly complete their work and prevent disease. It's been recommended to wash your hands after activities such as using the bathroom or working out and before eating.

Either way, the hand sanitizer is a great addition to the hygiene routine to prevent the spread of the new viruses and a great addition to the workplace to ensure employee's health.

Perhaps, it is possible to prepare hand sanitizers at home using cost-effective and quality products. As the hand sanitizers contain alcohol and other anti-bacterial and anti-viral disinfectants, they are effective in preventing the contraction of the germ and bacterial.

Since markets are running out of hand sanitizers, it is imperative to learn and try the homemade recipes to prepare quality alternatives at home. In this way, you get to know the ingredients of your sanitizers without blindly relying on the company manufactured products, and you can get to use your favorite scents and liquids along with alcohol. Your hand sanitizer can smell like lemons or lavender; now, it is all in your hand. So, give this book a read and refill your hand sanitizer bottles with a homemade quality product.

Professionals in the medical field invented hand sanitizers. Doctors and nurses need to keep their hands free of bacteria and germs. They need to avoid spreading them from one patient to the next. The sanitizer was discovered in the mid-1900s, and they come in the form of a gel. Since these products contain alcohol, they can dry your skin. It is for this reason that most people avoid using store-bought sanitizers. If you are one such person, you will prefer to make hand sanitizers at home.

Many claims that the alcohol component in most hand sanitizers can harm our skin-and this is valid to some degree. So much use is likely to dry the skin of our hands-so we should still use a lotion to prevent our hands from looking and feeling cold. This will also be assured that we use a sanitizer not just for our hands but even for items we use and handle daily, such as a keyboard, telephone, handbags, and also our mobile phones. According to a recent Fox News report, on the bottom of our bags, there are more bacteria than on our toilet seat. Unfortunately, e-coli and other forms of bacteria were found on the bottom of our luggage, since they have been placed almost everywhere, including on public bathroom floors.

Homemade hand sanitizer does not contain triclosan or other antibacterial agents. By using essential oils, you will inhibit bacteria naturally, always being careful to choose ones that are safe for kids. There is also some evidence that these oils can help eliminate viruses and bacteria, making them potentially more effective.

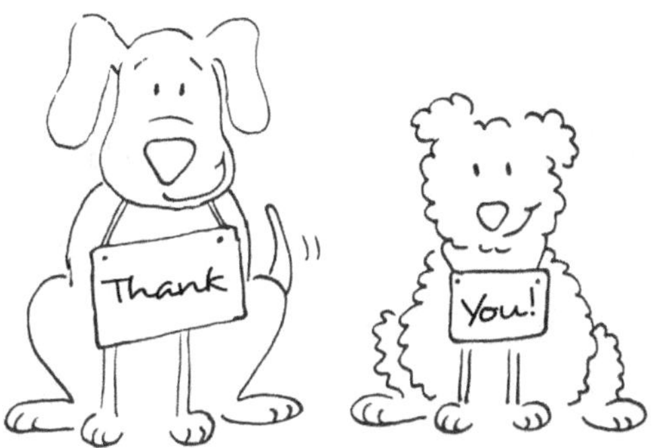

Thank You For Reading My Book !

First of all, thank you for purchasing this book .

I know you could have picked any number of books to read, but

you picked this book and for that I am extremely grateful.

I hope that it added at value and quality to your everyday life.

If so, it would be really nice if you could share this book with your

*friends and family by posting to **Facebook** and **Twitter** .*

If you enjoyed this book and found some benefit in reading this,

I'd like to hear from you and hope that you could take some time to

post a review on Amazon. Your feedback and support will help this

author to greatly improve his writing craft for future projects and

make this book even bette

By the Same Author

EMMA KINGS

HOME MADE
MEDICAL
FACE MASK

A BEGINNER'S GUIDE TO MAKE YOUR OWN DIY
REUSABLE AND WASHABLE PROTECTIVE FACE MASK
AT HOME IN FEW MINUTES WITH BASIC
HOUSEHOLD ITEMS

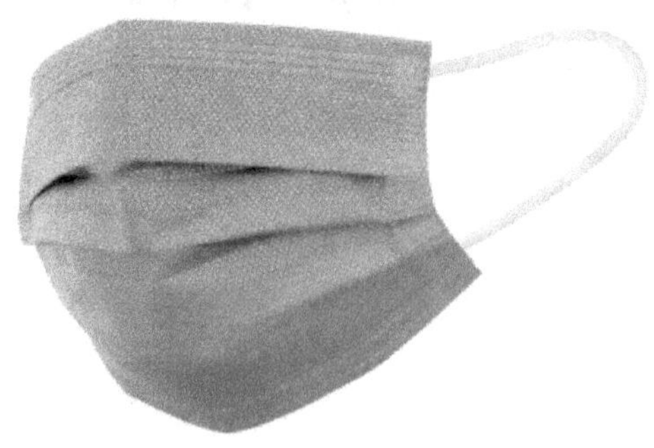

9 798640 617566